MASTERS OF HEALTH

The original sources of
today's alternative therapies

EDITED BY
ROBERT VAN DE WEYER

Copyright © 2005 O Books
O Books is an imprint of John Hunt Publishing Ltd., The Bothy,
Deershot Lodge, Park Lane, Ropley, Hants, SO24 0BE, UK
office@johnhunt-publishing.com
www.O-books.net

Distribution in:
UK
Orca Book Services
orders@orcabookservices.co.uk
Tel: 01202 665432 Fax: 01202 666219 Int. code (44)

USA and Canada
NBN
custserv@nbnbooks.com
Tel: 1 800 462 6420 Fax: 1 800 338 4550

Australia
Brumby Books
sales@brumbybooks.com
Tel: 61 3 9761 5535 Fax: 61 3 9761 7095

New Zealand
Peaceful Living
books@peaceful-living.co.nz
Tel: 64 7 57 18105 Fax: 64 7 57 18513

Singapore
STP
davidbuckland@tlp.com.sg
Tel: 65 6276 Fax: 65 6276 7119

South Africa
Alternative Books
altbook@global.co.za
Tel: 27 011 792 7730 Fax: 27 011 972 7787

Text: © 2005 Robert Van de Weyer

Design: BookDesign™, London

ISBN 1 905047 15 0

All rights reserved. Except for brief quotations in critical articles
or reviews, no part of this book may be reproduced in any manner
without prior written permission from the publishers.

The rights of Robert Van de Weyer as author and illustrator
respectively has/have been asserted in accordance with the
Copyright, Designs and Patents Act 1988.

A CIP catalogue record for this book is available from the British
Library.

Printed in the USA by Maple-Vail Manufacturing Group

MASTERS OF HEALTH

The original sources of
today's alternative therapies

EDITED BY
ROBERT VAN DE WEYER

BOOKS

WASHINGTON, USA
WINCHESTER, UK

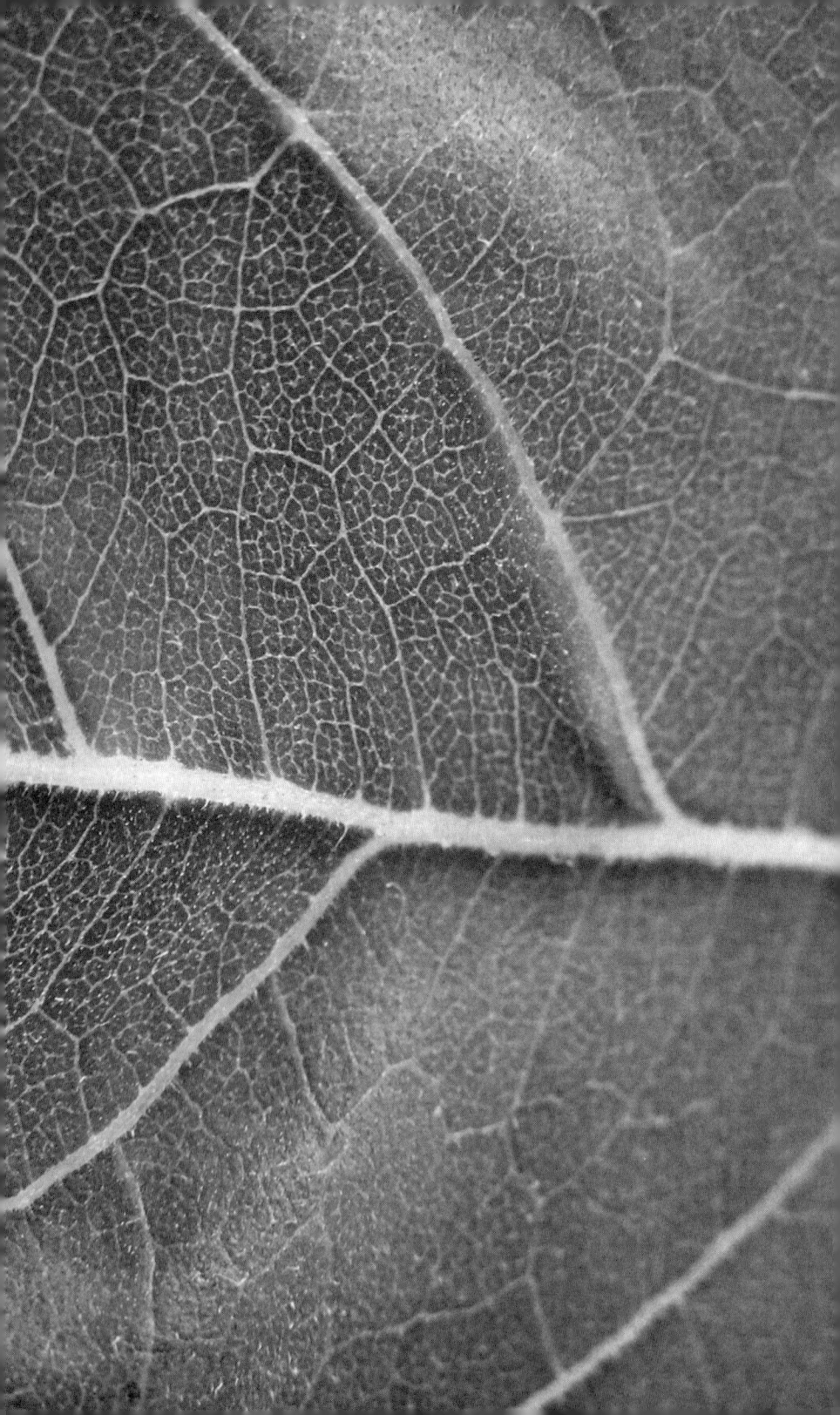

CONTENTS

General Introduction — 7

Huang Di	Yin and yang	9
Ayurveda	The science of life	27
Hippocrates	Self-treatment	39
Pliny	Plants as medicines	57
Raja Yoga	Discipline of the mind	65
Hatha Yoga	Discipline of the body	79
Tantra	The fabric of health	97
T'ai Chi	Health through movement	109
Muhammad	Simplicity and balance	129
Razi	Spiritual medicine	147
Hildegard	Body and soul	159
Andrew Boorde	Health through mirth	169

GENERAL INTRODUCTION

In the past century the average length of life in most western countries has approximately doubled; but the period of good health has increased much more slowly, and in recent decades appears to have stopped growing. Thus human beings now spend far more years suffering poor health and chronic illness than even before; and western medicine seems almost powerless to prevent this.

As a result there has been growing interest in alternative approaches to health and illness, especially those that have been tried and tested over many centuries and millennia. A majority of people in western countries now consult practitioners of alternative therapies from time to time; and numerous books describing these therapies have been published. But the original texts are hard to find, and remain largely unread; and some may wonder how true the modern books and practitioners are to the ancient ways.

Here are original texts from twelve approaches to health and illness that have proved their worth over a long period. In some cases the whole text has been given; in other cases the more technical parts have been left out.

Although these texts come from almost every part of the globe, there is a remarkable degree of unanimity about what constitutes a healthy way of life. Each text has some specific insights and prescriptions of its own; but generally these complement, rather than conflict with, the insights and prescriptions of the others. Thus taken together these twelve texts form a summary of ancient wisdom on human wholeness, and when we compare here the remedies of 21st-century therapists, we can see how faithful they are to the well tried remedies of the past.

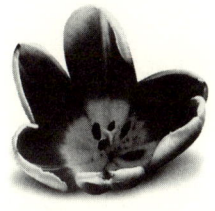

Huang Di

Yin and Yang

INTRODUCTION

Huang Di's *Book of Internal Medicine* **is probably the oldest book on** health and healing that exists; parts of it may have been composed over four thousand years ago. Its approach to health and healing is based on the principles of Yin and Yang, which are central to much Chinese philosophy and religion. And it contains the earliest exposition of the art of acupuncture, and also of moxa – a practice that involves placing a mixture of herbs on the skin and lighting it.

Huang Di, the 'Yellow Emperor', is supposed to have lived around 2600 BCE. According to legend he was a man of great ingenuity, inventing the wheel, the ship, and soldiers' armor. Since there are no contemporary documents or archeological remains testifying to his activities, some modern historians question his existence. Moreover, the book's lack of structure and its frequent repetition suggest that it grew over a long period, with successive authors adding their own insights. But regardless of its true authorship the book attributed to Huang Di remains the basis of Chinese medicine; and its methods of treatment are now used across the globe.

Yin and Yang broadly correspond to the female and the male principles of Nature. Yang stands for sunlight, fire, heat, and dryness; Yin stands for moonlight, earth, coolness and moisture. Yang is active and constantly moving, while Yin is passive and still. In terms of human temperament Yang represent exuberance and joy, while Yin represents melancholy and sadness. The essence of good health, according to Huang Di, is to maintain balance between Yin and Yang.

CHAPTER 1

THE UNIVERSAL PRINCIPLE

The principle of Yin and Yang is the basic principle of the entire universe. It is the root and source of life and death. In order to treat and cure diseases one must understand this principle.

Obedience to the laws of Yin and Yang means life; disobedience means death. Obedience brings harmony and order; disobedience brings confusion and disorder.

Yang is the element of light. The essences of Yang unite and ascend to the sky, creating clarity and light above. Yin is the element of darkness. The essences of Yin unite and descend to earth, creating fullness and abundance below.

Yin is active inside the body, and regulates Yang. Yang is active on the outside of the body, and regulates Yin. When Yang is too strong, the body becomes hot, and the person starts to pant; the mouth becomes dry, and the bowels become constipated. For a person in such a condition the heat of summer is unendurable. When Yin is too strong, the body becomes cold, and the limbs start to tremble; the stomach cannot digest food properly, so the person suffers diarrhea. For a person in such a condition the cold of winter is unendurable.

Yin stores up the essences within the body, and prepares them for use. Yang uses those essences, protecting the body from external danger. If

Yin is less than Yang, the pulse becomes weak, the body sickly, and the mind confused. If Yang is less than Yin, the internal organs conflict with one another, and the orifices become blocked. Thus wise people keep Yin and Yang in balance. They eat appropriately to ensure the pulse and the muscles are in harmony; they exercise in order to make their bones and marrow strong; and they breathe deeply and steadily. By keeping Yin and Yang in balance the eyes remain clear, the ears remain alert, and the mind remains sharp. Thus the life force is kept in its original, pristine state.

People with passive temperaments are primarily influenced by Yin; people with active temperaments are primarily influenced by Yang. Those influenced by Yin are slow and dilatory, and are more prone to diseases of the internal organs. Those influenced by Yang are quick and energetic, and are more prone to diseases of the external organs.

When Yin is excessive, and thus overwhelming Yang, the person will have terrifying dreams of wading or swimming, and almost drowning. When Yang is excessive, and thus overwhelming Yin, the person will have terrifying dreams of being caught in fires, and almost burning to death. When Yin and Yang are both strong, but in conflict, the person will have dreams of fighting and warfare.

If people are to be free of disease and to enjoy good health, they must want Yin and Yang to be in harmony. The wise healer only treats people who have this desire.

We all know men who constantly assert their own wills, and who are ceaselessly active; and we know women who constantly submit to the will of others, preferring the safety of passivity. Huang Di teaches that the macho man and the mousy woman are actually endangering their health, since they are suppressing one part of themselves – they are leading unbalanced lives. So are we simultaneously aware of the active and the passive tendencies within us, and do we allow both to express themselves? The kind of minor ailments to which we are prone, and the kind of dreams which we can remember having, may offer clues.

CHAPTER 2

THE INTERNAL AND EXTERNAL ORGANS

The organs of the human body relating to the outside world are Yang; the internal organs are Yin. There are five internal organs belonging to Yin: liver, heart, pancreas, lungs and kidneys. There are five external organs belonging to Yang: gall-bladder, stomach, intestines, urinary bladder and skin.

The heart is the root of life, and thus controls the spiritual faculties. It fills the pulse with blood, and influences the face. The complexion of a person reveals the condition of the heart.

The lungs are the origin of breath, and are where spirit of a person is located. They are connected with the skin and the hair. The sheen of a person's hair reveals the condition of the lungs.

The liver is the source of energy, and is where the spirit relates to the universal spirit. It is connected with the muscles, and the nails. The state of a person's finger and toenails, and the amount of energy a person has, reveal the condition of the liver.

The kidneys are where the vital essences are stored. They are connected with the bones. The strength and hardness of a person's bones reveal the condition of the kidneys.

The pancreas is the source of transformation, enabling a person to change from good to evil, or evil to good. The pancreas is connected with the flesh. The color of a person's lips reveals the condition of the pancreas.

The head is the home of skill and intelligence. When the head is constantly bowed, so the person is only looking down, eventually the spirit will be broken.

The back is the main wall of the home where all the internal organs reside. When the back is constantly bent, through carrying heavy burdens, the internal organs will be crushed.

If the breath is too plentiful, this indicates that disease is likely to occur in the external organs. If breath is too little, this indicates that disease has reached the internal organs.

Although we cannot be directly aware of the organs mentioned by Huang Di, except the skin, we can make ourselves aware of all the symptoms of their functioning that he enumerates. And although we may not be convinced of all the connections he makes between organs and symptoms, we can distinguish between good and bad symptoms. So are we checking from time to time the quality of our complexion, hair, nails, lips, posture, breath and so on? And if the quality is poor, are we honest and brave enough to confront those aspects of our daily life that may be wrong? Much of the rest of Huang Di's teaching indicates the kind of changes that we may need to make.

CHAPTER 3

EMOTIONS

There are five emotions: joy, anger, sympathy, grief and fear. If one of these emotions becomes dominant, the spirit is injured, causing severe spiritual pain. This may in time injure the internal organs, causing physical illness.

Extreme joy may injure the heart. Extreme anger injures the liver. Extreme sympathy injures the pancreas. Extreme grief injures the lungs. Extreme fear injures the kidneys and bowels.

The antidote to joy is fear; to anger is sympathy; to sympathy is anger; to grief is joy; to fear is contemplation.

When a person too frequently becomes angry or frightened, the force of Yang overwhelms Yin. Ulcers appear on the skin and on the internal organs. The orifices, especially the nose and throat, are liable to become blocked. The person can also suffer flatulence and intermittent fevers; and the complexion becomes red.

Wise people learn to prevent this happening. But if it does occur, the person should try to dissipate the excess Yang through rest and relaxation. Acupuncture may assist in removing blockages that have formed, allowing the excess Yang to drain away.

When there is an excess of joy, the person will dream of flying. When there is an excess of grief, the person will dream of falling down. When there is an excess of anger, the person will dream of violence. When there is an excess of sympathy, the person will dream of gliding through water like a fish. When there is an excess of fear, the person will dream of having insects buzzing around.

The healer should seek to open the mind and hearts of patients, and let them express their feelings. Those who can express interest in the people and things around them, and possess a sense of purpose, are likely to overcome their illness. Those who can find no interest in people and things, and have lost all sense of purpose, are likely to be overcome by their illness.

All of us are aware that too much anger or fear is both uncomfortable in itself, and also physically damaging; very hot-tempered or anxious people often look unhealthy, and are more prone to both minor and major illnesses. But have we ever wondered whether we can suffer from too much sympathy for others, or too much joy? Huang Di teaches that these apparently positive emotions, when experienced in excess, are just as dangerous as negative emotions. Moreover, in order to control the negative emotions, we must also limit the positive ones. Huang Di is cautioning us against intense feelings of all kinds, and inviting us to be serene.

CHAPTER 4

TIMES AND SEASONS

At dawn the breath of Yang is activated; at midday the breath of Yang is at its most abundant; as the sun moves to the west, the breath of Yang declines; when the sun sets, the breath of Yang can again barely be discerned. The breath of Yang warms the flesh and loosens the muscles, enabling the muscles to work well. If the flesh is exposed to the cold mists and dews of the night, the muscles become rigid, and their strength is lost.

The three months of spring are the period when life begins and is renewed. In spring people should rise early; they should first have a brisk walk, and then a leisurely stroll. During spring people should be gentle with their bodies; they should give their bodies rewards, not punishments. Those defying the laws of spring will suffer injury to the liver; and in summer they will catch chills.

The three months of summer are the period of luxuriant growth. In summer people should rise early. As the heat of the day intensifies, they should be careful not to weary themselves; and they should not allow themselves to become angry. During summer people should concentrate on developing the best features of both their minds and their bodies. Through breathing deeply, they should bring the outside world deep within their bodies. They should love every aspect of the outside world. Those defying the laws of summer will suffer injury to the heart; and in the fall they will feel weak, unable to stand the colder weather.

The three months of the fall are the period of tranquility. In the fall people should retire early at night, and rise in the morning with the crowing of the rooster. They should keep their minds peaceful. During the fall people should not give expression to their physical desires; they should turn inwards, and concentrate on their souls. They should beware of breathing air that is foul or impure. Those defying the laws of the fall will suffer injury to the lungs; and in winter they will be prone to indigestion and diarrhea.

The three months of winter are the period of death in life. In winter people should retire early at night, and rise late with the rising of the sun. They should try to escape the cold and seek warmth; yet from time to time they should breathe in the cold air.

During winter people should suppress and conceal their desires, as if all their wishes had already been fulfilled. They should not try to achieve anything, freeing their hearts from any urge to assert their will. Those defying the laws of winter will suffer injury to the kidneys and testicles; and in spring they will be impotent.

The interaction of the four seasons and the interaction of Yin and Yang is the foundation of everything in the world. Wise people nurture and develop their Yang in spring and summer, and nurture and develop their Yin in the fall and spring. Those failing to do this sever their own roots, causing themselves to wither and die.

Those injured in the summer by heat will suffer intermittent fever in the fall. Those injured in the fall through humidity will suffer cough and impotence in the winter. Those injured in the winter through extreme cold will be weak and slow in the spring.

Exposure of the body to extreme cold induces intense heat in the form of fevers. Exposure of the body to intense heat induces extreme cold in the form of chills.

If people try to hurry in the heat of summer, or they become angry, they start to pant furiously, and sweat pours from them. And when they calm down, their minds are confused. Their bodies resemble burning charcoal. In this situation they must rest quietly, allowing the perspiration to carry away the fever. But if they persist in their folly, their Yang becomes exhausted, the orifices of the body become blocked, and they may even cease to sweat. They will then collapse, and it may be impossible to halt the onset of death.

In an age of electric light at the flick of a switch, we can virtually ignore the natural rhythm of the day and the night; night only comes when we turn off the lights. And in an age of central heating at home, and air-conditioning in offices and shops, we can almost ignore the rhythm of the seasons. Yet the human body evolved to adapt and respond to these natural rhythms; and Huang Di describes these bodily responses. Are we listening to our bodies, and hearing what he describes; and are we modifying our behavior accordingly? Do we, for example, confine our most demanding activities to the early part of the day, so that we can gradually relax in the latter part? Do we rise earlier in the spring and summer, exercise more vigorously, and thence breathe more deeply?

CHAPTER 5

FOOD AND AIR

There are five flavors: sourness, saltiness, sweetness, bitterness and pungency. If sourness exceeds the other flavors, an excess of saliva and phlegm is produced, blocking the orifices. If saltiness exceeds the other flavors, the bones become weary, the heart becomes weak, and the mind anxious. If sweetness exceeds the other flavors, the lungs become breathless, the complexion darkens, and the kidneys become unbalanced. If bitterness exceeds the other flavors, the body becomes dry, and the stomach becomes heavy and upset. If pungency exceeds the other flavors, the muscles and the pulse become slack, and the mind depressed. It is important, therefore, to balance and mix the five flavors well. In this way the bones will remain straight, the muscles will remain tender, the breath will remain regular and deep, the blood will circulate freely, and the complexion will be clear.

When flavors are unbalanced in the food we eat, and one strong flavor dominates, the Yin is weakened. This allows the Yang to dominate. The result is that passions become excessively strong, exhausting the body and confusing the mind.

The heart craves bitter flavor; the lungs crave pungent flavor; the liver craves sour flavor; the stomach craves sweet flavor; the kidneys crave salt flavor. If the five flavors are correctly combined and balanced, all the internal organs will be satisfied and remain healthy.

Those with disease of the liver should eat only a little pungent food to prevent their liver from disintegrating, and sour food to drain the liver of excessive fullness. Those with disease of the heart should only eat a little salty food to make the heart pliable, and then sweet foods such as fruits to drain the heart of excessive fullness. Those with disease of the stomach should eat less than they desire; they should have only a little sweet food to set the stomach at ease, and then eat bitter food to drain the stomach of excessive fullness. Those with disease of the lungs should eat sour food to strengthen the lungs, and then pungent food to drain the lungs of excessive fullness. Those with disease of the kidneys should eat bitter food to strengthen the kidneys, and then salty food to drain the kidneys of excessive fullness.

In herbs we taste all the five flavors: bitterness, sourness, sweetness, pungency and saltiness. The five flavors can be perfectly balanced and blended by mixing the herbs correctly. Then, when they are eaten and stored in the stomach, they will spread a healthy atmosphere through the body and the mind.

When a disease of an internal organ begins, the person should consume only hot water and rice soup for ten days. Only after this period, if the disease is not yet cured, should medicines be taken. Diseases of the external organs do not require reduction in diet.

The different winds may induce different illnesses. The wind blowing from the sea causes problems to the throat, nose and neck. The opposite wind blowing from the land causes problems to the shoulder and back. The warm south wind can cause disturbance to the chest and ribs. The cold north wind can cause problems in the loins and thighs. So, depending on which way the wind is blowing, people should be gentle towards the parts of the body that are most vulnerable. Oppressive humid weather upsets the mind, causing madness. Constant wind upsets the stomach, making it unable to retain food and digest it. Frosty air causes ulcers.

With the discovery of vitamins, minerals and proteins in our food over the past century, we have become accustomed to the idea of a nutritionally balanced diet. But we now have the illusion that we understand fully the relationship between nutrition and health; so many of us consume a very unnatural diet, assuring ourselves that it has all the nutrients we need, and is therefore balanced. In fact new nutritional discoveries are constantly being made, suggesting that our ignorance may still exceed our knowledge. Huang Di draws our attention to our natural mechanism for achieving a balanced diet: our sense of taste. Do we overemphasize particular flavors in our diet because we especially like those flavors? And how can we modify our diet so that the different flavors are balanced? And when we've made those modifications, do they accord with our present scientific knowledge of healthy nutrition?

CHAPTER 6

PULSE AND COMPLEXION

If you want to understand illness, observe yourself. Learn to notice small changes in yourself, and see from experience how these are symptoms of internal disturbance.

The complexion and the pulse are the two most valuable means of discerning a person's condition. The complexion corresponds with the sun, the pulse with the moon. The complexion changes as the pulse changes; the one reflects the other.

The pulse should be taken at dawn when the breath of Yin has not yet begun to stir, and when the breath of Yang has not yet begun to diffuse; when food and drink have not yet been taken; and when energy has not yet been exerted.

A healthy person has one exhalation of breath to two pulse beats, and one inhalation of breath to two pulse beats. In spring the pulse should be fine and delicate like the strings of a musical instrument. In summer the pulse should be like the beats of a fine hammer. In the fall the pulse should be soft and gentle like a lullaby. In winter the pulse should be small and hard, like a stone.

When the pulse beats are very deep and thin, this indicates excess Yin in the body; the person will tend to suffer chills. When the pulse beats are hasty and panting, this indicates excess Yang in the body; the person will tend to suffer fevers. When the pulse beats are soft and scattered, yet the complexion is clear and shiny, this indicates the body is dehydrated; the person must drink more fluids. When the pulse beats are very quick, so that there are six beats to every cycle of breath, this indicates disease of the heart. When the pulse beat is very loud, this indicates disease of the pancreas. When the pulse beats are very full and slow, this indicates disease of the stomach; so the person is prone to indigestion. When the pulse beats are empty and slow, this indicates confusion of the brain. When the pulse beats are full and quick, this indicates the person is prone to headaches. When the pulse beats are large and heavy, this indicates disease of the kidneys.

If the complexion is red, this indicates evil influences in the heart; the diagnosis is confirmed if the person also suffers a persistent cough. If the complexion is pale, this indicates evil influence in the lungs; the diagnosis is confirmed if the person has a light cough and is short of breath. If the complexion has a green tinge, this indicates evil influence in the liver; the diagnosis is confirmed if there is lack of energy in the limbs, and if the feet hurt. If the complexion has a yellow tinge, this indicates evil influence in the pancreas; the diagnosis is confirmed in the person perspires excessively. If the complexion is gray and dark, this indicates evil influence in the kidneys; the diagnosis is confirmed if the person is restless.

Many of us are so accustomed, even addicted, to stress that we barely notice how stressed we are. Yet there is ample evidence that a high level of stress reduces our immunity, and in the long term makes us more vulnerable to heart disease and even cancer. And part of our addiction to stress that we cannot even slow down during our hours off work, but must be equally frenetic in our leisure. The pulse and the complexion, Huang Di's favored means of diagnosis, are ideal for monitoring this modern plague. As he suggests, we should check the pulse as we wake in the morning, when we are most relaxed – and then check it at odd moments through the day. And we should check the complexion soon after rising, when signs of unhealthy living are most visible. Is the pulse racing through much of the day, and even the evening? And is the 'morning face' a horror to behold? We ignore these simple signs at our peril.

CHAPTER 7

ACUPUNCTURE AND MOXA

Those wishing to practice acupuncture should meditate frequently in silence. They should be honest and generous in word and action. They should know the difference between beauty and ugliness.

The purpose of acupuncture is to supply what is lacking, and to drain off excess. When the needle is applied to places that are hollow and empty, those places will be replenished. When the needle is applied to places that are full and solid, those places will be drained.

Experts in acupuncture follow the principle of Yin to draw out Yang; and they follow the principle of Yang to draw out Yin. They use the right hand to treat illnesses on the left side; and they use the left hand to treat illnesses on the right side.

When the pulse is beating strongly, the healer should apply moxa in the area of Yin, and needles of acupuncture in the area of Yang. When the pulse is weak, the healer should apply the needles of acupuncture in the area of Yang, and moxa in the area of Yin.

The wise healer is capable of applying every type of treatment: acupuncture with flint needles and with metal needles; herbal medicines; moxa; and massage. The healer should diagnose each patient, and then apply the appropriate combination of these treatments.

When a person's body is balanced and content, but the mind and emotions are in distress, cure the distress by using both moxa treatment and acupuncture. When a person's body is balanced and content, when the emotions are tranquil, but when the mind is in distress, use acupuncture only. When a person's body is balanced and content, when the mind is tranquil, but when the emotions are in distress, use moxa and breathing exercises. When a person's body is ill, and when the mind and emotions are in distress, use acupuncture, moxa, breathing exercises and herbal medicine.

The human being has three hundred and sixty-five small ducts. These protect the life force, and prevent evil influences from entering. When acupuncture is applied correctly to these ducts, it causes evil influences to depart.

The needle should be inserted when the patient is inhaling. The needle should be left for a while, and the patient should breathe quietly. The needle should be turned a little when the patient is inhaling. The needle should be taken out when the patient is exhaling; it should be withdrawn slowly, and only come out completely when the patient has completely exhaled.

When acupuncture does not cure a disease immediately, it should be repeated. The needle should be applied quietly and with the utmost care.

Faith in any particular treatment helps the treatment to work. Yet we should initially be skeptical of all treatments, since many treatments, which were once hailed as miraculous, have later turned out to have damaging long-term effects that may outweigh any short-term benefits. Finding the right balance, in relation to medicine, between faith and doubt is extremely hard. But when a treatment has been used over many centuries and even millennia, and has been found to be often beneficial and never harmful, then faith is justified. Acupuncture meets those criteria. So, for those ailments that acupuncture claims to help, why not use it?

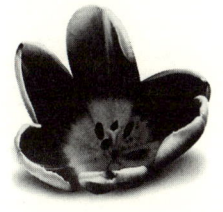

Ayurveda

THE SCIENCE OF LIFE

INTRODUCTION

Ayu means 'life', and *veda* means 'knowledge' or 'science'. So Ayurveda is the 'science of life'.

The two main texts of Ayurveda, the *Charaka Samhita* and the *Sushrata Samhita*, were both written in the late second millennium BCE, at about the same time as the main Hindu scriptures, the *Vedas*. And like the *Vedas*, they were based on knowledge that had been handed down orally for many centuries previously. By the middle of the first millennium Ayurvedic physicians were common throughout northern India.

Ayurvedic medicine was greatly boosted by the growth of Buddhism. An Ayurvedic physician called Jivaka was an early disciple of the Buddha; and the Buddha himself benefited from his treatment. And when in c3 BCE the emperor of northern India, Ashoka, converted to Buddhism, he introduced Ayurvedic hospitals throughout his territories, treating animals as well as humans.

The Ayurvedic texts have medical prescriptions for every illness; and the physician must train for many years to become familiar with them all. But the basic principles of Ayurveda are quite simple; and its advice about daily life is directed to everyone. Each of the texts comprises several volumes; the following pieces are taken from the *Sushrata Samhita*.

CHAPTER I

PHILOSOPHICAL PRINCIPLES

Ayurveda has three aims: to treat disease, to maintain good health, and to prolong life.

It consists of knowledge that has been acquired by three methods: observation of human health and disease; inference drawn from what has been observed; and analogy, in which similar causes are regarded as having similar effects.

Disease is defined as any kind of suffering in a human being.

The technological progress of the West has depended on the scientific method, which consists of testing ideas and observing results; and this is how modern western medicine developed. Ayurvedic medicine, which predates western science by almost two millennia, is also founded on the scientific method of testing and observing. So if we are willing to consume the pills produced by modern drug companies, why should we not be equally willing to consult an Ayurvedic physician?

CHAPTER 2

THE NATURE OF DISEASE

Human beings have three aspects or humors: wind, bile and phlegm. When these three humors are in equilibrium, the person is healthy. But when they are out of balance, disease occurs. All diseases are caused by imbalance of the humors.

The humors interact with the seven types of tissue: plasma, blood, muscle, fat, bone, bone marrow, and semen. They also interact with the three excreta: stool, urine, and sweat. When there is imbalance in the humors, damage occurs in the tissues, and the process of excretion become blocked.

If there is excess wind, the voice is hoarse, the skin is dark and liable to twitch, the bowels are constipated, the body is cold, and the patient has difficulty sleeping. If there is deficient wind, the patient is sluggish, listless and discontented.

If there is excess bile, the skin and the eyes are yellow, the stool is also yellow, the senses are dull, the body is hot, and the patient frequently feels faint. If there is deficient bile, the patient is cold, and has poor digestion.

If there is excess phlegm, the skin is pale, the limbs are stiff and weak, the digestion is poor, breathing is difficult, and the patient sleeps too long. If there is deficient phlegm, the body and mouth are dry, the joints are loose, and the patient has difficulty sleeping.

There are seven groups of diseases: hereditary diseases, which may be transmitted through the father or the mother; diseases caused by improper care before birth; diseases caused by the wrong diet and daily routine; injury; seasonal diseases; diseases caused by evil spirits; and natural diseases caused by hunger, thirst and old age.

Some diseases can be cured completely. Some diseases can be relieved: their symptoms are reduced, while the disease remains. Some diseases can be neither cured nor relieved.

We have come to expect that the normal human condition is freedom from disease; and drug companies invest huge amounts of money in finding pills for every ill. Ayurveda urges us to abandon this expectation. And experience suggests that Ayurveda is right: modern medicine has helped us to live longer; but we remain beset by numerous chronic conditions for which no complete cure is likely to be discovered. What, then, is our attitude to illness? We are pleased to be cured of those diseases that are curable, and relieved of those symptoms that can be alleviated. But do we allow our chronic conditions to become curses over our lives? Or can we find ways of accepting them serenely, and even perhaps even turning them into blessings? In learning to cope with physical discomfort or disability, we may become kinder and gentler, both to others and to ourselves.

CHAPTER 3

DIAGNOSIS AND TREATMENT

The physician examines the patient through each of the senses. Examination by eye shows the patient's state of nourishment, and the color of the skin. Examination by touch shows whether the patient's body is hot or cold, whether the patient's skin is rough or smooth, and whether the patient's flesh is hard or soft. Examination by ear, pressed against the flesh, can show where any blockages occur. Examination by taste shows disorders in the urine. And examination by smell can show the presence of ulcers.

In diagnosing a disease the physician should take into account the age and location of the patient. Excess wind is most common is dry areas, and amongst the old. Excess bile is most common in dry areas, and amongst adults. Excess phlegm is most common in swampy areas and amongst the young.

There are four methods of treatment: use of drugs; change of diet; and massage. In determining the correct program of treatment the physician must consider three factors: the nature of the patient; the nature of the disease; and the season of the year.

Modern physicians, when prescribing treatment, tend to concentrate on the nature of the disease; their training, and the constraints of time, do not encourage consideration of the particular nature of the patient, let alone such extraneous factors as the season. Yet a treatment for a particular disease may be effective for one patient, and useless or harmful to another – suggesting that the nature of the patient is crucial. The person likely to know a patient best is, of course, the patient; and many of us have intuitions about the treatments that physicians prescribe to us. Ayurveda suggests that we should listen carefully to those intuitions; and if we intuitively feel a particular treatment is wrong for us, we should have the courage to resist it.

CHAPTER 4

DIET

To maintain health and cure disease, it is important to be the correct weight. Overweight people are liable to suffer excess bile; and all diseases are worsened by excess fat. Underweight people are liable to suffer nervous disorders; and all diseases are made worse by lack of fat.

Cereals are central to a healthy diet. Rice is the easiest cereal to digest, and tends to cool the body; so it is good for patients with excess bile. Wheat slows down the process of ageing, helps to heal wounds, and is a laxative; it is good for patients with excess wind.

Meat from animals that run swiftly, like deer, strengthens the heart and bladder, and is good for patients with excess wind and bile. Meat from animals that like swampy conditions, like pigs, and from ducks helps wounds to heal quickly, and is good for patients with excess phlegm. The flesh of the female is better than that of the male in curing diseases – except birds, where the flesh of the male is preferable. The liver is the most nutritious part of any animal, with the greatest healing power.

Fruits with a sharp taste, such as pomegranate, are good for the heart; and they are good for patients with deficient wind. Mangoes improve the complexion, help the blood to flow, and loosen the limbs. Coconuts, bananas and grapes are laxatives, they improve the voice, and they help bring down fevers. Fruits should only be eaten when they are ripe.

Garlic has great value in curing and preventing illness. It is a laxative, it increases semen, it improves memory, it strengthens the voice, it clears the complexion, it enables the eyes to focus more precisely, it helps fractured bones to unite, it cures heart disease and piles, it brings down fevers, it eases swelling of the belly, it relieves coughs, it improves the digestion, it reduces asthma, and it expels worms.

Honey has the greatest value of all foods in curing and preventing illness. There is no disease that honey will not help to cure.

Milk, especially from goats, is good for chest diseases. Yogurt is good for all diseases, and helps to prevent illness; it should be made from cow's milk.

Food should be eaten in a place that is both clean and quiet; and meals should never be hurried. Sweet food should be consumed first, followed by salty and sour foods.

Most nutritional judgments of foods today are based on chemical analyses of the calories, proteins, carbohydrates, fats, fiber, vitamins and minerals they contain. But there remains considerable uncertainty about the desirable levels for each of us to consume of these things; there may be many other nutrients of which we are barely aware; and different people may have quite different nutritional needs. Ayurvedic nutritional judgments are based on simple observations of the effects of each food; and these observations take into account different people's conditions. So in what do we put our trust, chemical analysis or empirical observation? Happily Ayurvedic guidance does not conflict with modern nutritional chemistry, and to a great degree is confirmed by it. And certainly the Ayurvedic advice about the desirable context for eating is undoubtedly wise – and is wholly at odds with today's fast food culture.

CHAPTER 5

SLEEP, EXERCISE AND SEX

Sleep should occur in a comfortable bed. The bedroom should be free of all draughts.

Adequate sleep brings health, happiness and a long life. Difficulty in sleeping, or excessive sleeping, is a sign of disease. Difficulty in sleeping can be eased by massage, and by sweet foods. Excessive sleeping can be overcome by a period of fasting, followed by a permanent reduction in the amount of food eaten.

Dreams foretell the outcome of an illness. If, for example, a patient dreams of riding an elephant, the outcome is likely to be good. But if a patient dreams of falling off a mountain or being eaten by crows, then death is the likely outcome.

Exercise is vital to good health. It reduces fat and increases strength. A person should exercise each day until the breath becomes rapid and the body breaks into a sweat.

Excessive sexual intercourse induces disease, while suppression of the sexual urge promotes good health and longevity. Young men and women may safely have intercourse once every two or three days in winter, but only once a fortnight in summer and during rainy weather. Semen should never be retained when it is on the point of discharge.

There have been numerous theories about the nature of sleep and the meaning of dreams, and almost as many about the relationship between sexual activity and physical health. These theories contradict one another, and none is proven – and perhaps proof is impossible. Yet we each have intuitions on these matters: we know when we are sleeping too little or two much; we often gain valuable insights from our dreams about our own deeper feelings; and our emotions, as well as our bodies, tell us when sex is right and wrong. Ayurveda may help stimulate our intuition. When we seem chronically tired, why not try reducing our intake of food? When we lie awake tossing and turning, rather than turn to pills, why not try some systematic technique for relaxation? And if in certain seasons our libido diminishes, why not be content with a time of celibacy? But on one thing everyone agrees: vigorous exercise at least once a day is highly beneficial.

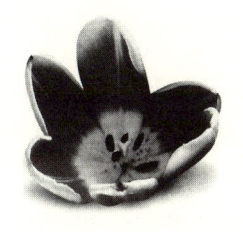

Hippocrates

SELF-TREATMENT

INTRODUCTION

Hippocrates is credited with turning the healer's art from a form of magic to a science, based on experiment and observation; thus he is revered as the founder of western medicine. Yet he advised people to be wary both of drugs and physicians; and he urged them to treat themselves, both to maintain health and to cure sickness. Thus he could equally be regarded as the founder of alternative medicine.

Almost nothing is known for certain about his life; and some even doubt his existence, regarding the corpus of work credited to him as the collected writings of a school of medical philosophy. However, both Plato and Aristotle recognized him both as real and as a genius. According to them he was born on the island of Cos early in c5 BCE; he practiced as a physician throughout the Greek-speaking world, traveling from place to place; and he died at the age of 90.

Hippocrates distinguished two kinds of illness: those that many people contract at the same time, and are therefore carried through the air; and those that individuals contract, and are mainly caused by their particular circumstances and way of life. His main interest was illnesses of the second kind, and he tried to show how they could be prevented and cured by quite simple changes to diet, environment and daily routine.

CHAPTER I

PRINCIPLES OF HEALING

Good health is your most precious possession. Thus you should learn how to treat your own illnesses.

Some diseases are caused by the manner of life that you lead; others by the air you breathe. When there is an epidemic, the cause is clearly something common to all; and this must be in the air they breathe. But when many different diseases appear at the same time, clearly the cause lies in each individual's pattern of life.

A disease caused by your pattern of life should be treated by the opposite of its cause. Thus the cure for diseases caused by over-eating is fasting; the cure for diseases caused by starvation is feeding up. The cure for diseases caused by excessive exertion is rest; the cure for those caused by indolence is exertion.

It is dangerous to make sudden changes in your diet or in any other aspect of life. All sudden changes are inimical to human nature. Thus when you change their diet or some other aspect of life for the sake of your health, proceed gradually little by little.

Use drugs only very seldom, and then at the early stage of a disease. Before using drugs, ensure that you fully understand the disease, so that you can be sure which drugs are appropriate. When a disease has reached its crisis, or when the crisis has just passed, do not disturb your body with drugs or stimulants; let yourself recover naturally.

In every disease a healthy state of mind and a good appetite is beneficial. But if you allow yourself to become depressed, or to lose interest in food, the disease is likely to get worse.

Of all organs the brain is most sensitive to environmental factors, because it perceives its environment directly through the five senses. Thus an unhealthy environment and sudden changes in the environment tend to cause mental problems. The cure for diseases of the mind must, therefore, be sought in the environment; healing comes through making the right environmental changes.

Hippocrates is often described as the father of western medicine; yet his principles of healing strike at the heart of many of our medical attitudes. Are we not too prone to trust in experts, rather than in our own judgments? Do we not too often shun the obvious and simple cure for our ills, preferring something more complicated and supposedly more scientific? Do we not subject ourselves too often to drastic slimming diets or food fads, instead of making gradual improvements to our eating habits? Are we not liable to take occasional vigorous exercise, such as skiing or surfing, instead of taking moderate exercise daily? Do we not reach immediately for a drug when illness strikes, and thereby possibly interfere with the body's natural powers of healing? And when illnesses are chronic, or frequently recurring, how ready are we to question the environment in which we live or work?

CHAPTER 2

DIET AND EXERCISE

Food and exercise possess opposite qualities, yet together they promote good health. Exercise uses up energy, while food and drink replenish it. You should find those forms of exercise best suited to your body; and you should adjust the amount of food they eat to the amount of exercise you take.

The power of foods to disturb the body, or to promote harmony, is affected by the way in which they are prepared. Strong foods should be boiled. Moist foods should be grilled or roasted. Dry foods should be soaked and boiled, as should very salty foods. Bitter and sharp foods should be mixed with sweet ones. Astringent foods should be mixed with oily ones. Food should always be fresh, rather than stale.

During winter you should eat more and drink less. Your wine should be mixed with only a little water. You should eat bread rather than barley-cake; meat and fish should be roasted; and vegetables should be well cooked. This diet will keep your body warm and dry.

When spring comes, you should eat less and drink more. You should dilute your wine with a greater amount of water. You should eat fewer cereals, and substitute barley-cake for bread. Meat should be reduced, and it should be boiled rather than roasted. More vegetables should be eaten, and some may be eaten raw. This change should happen gradually as the atmosphere becomes warmer.

During summer the barley-cake should be soft and moist, all meat should be boiled, many raw vegetables should be eaten, and wine diluted with large amounts of water. This will keep the body cool and moist.

When the fall comes, this process should be reversed, until the winter diet is resumed.

Food may be salty, bitter, sweet, sharp, astringent, and fatty. When these qualities are properly mixed and balanced in a food, it is nutritious. But when one quality is dominant, the food will cause harm. In general, the various qualities are best mixed and balanced in simple foods.

Some like to dine once a day, and so make this their habit. Others prefer to eat twice, once at noon and again in the evening. It makes little difference to most your health whether you have one meal a day or two. But if you do not keep a regular pattern of eating, you are liable to become ill, and you will also find it difficult to sleep. If for some reason you are compelled to have a meal at an unusual time, you should rest afterwards.

When you are sick, do not alter your diet to any great extent, as this will upset you; simply eat less. You may also turn your normal food into a gruel in order that you can digest it more easily.

You may be tempted to eat too much; and when you start to overeat, the symptoms are pleasant. You sleep longer at night, and may also sleep more during the day, because their body is moist and restful. But soon the surfeit of food disturbs both your body and your soul. You no longer feel relaxed, and you frequently wake during the night; and your dreams become nasty and frightening. You feel aches in your flesh, as if you had over-exerted yourself; and, deluding yourself that you are indeed exercising too much, you may become even more indolent and self-indulgent. You may also bathe too frequently, in order to ease the aches; and excessive bathing combined with overeating can cause pneumonia. A further symptom is that after sexual intercourse you feel utterly exhausted, barely able to move.

It is vital to reduce your intake of food before pneumonia and other serious diseases attack. You may eat bread that is still warm, and vegetables such as leeks and onions; but you should have little meat. You should also eat only once a day, preferably in the evening. You should take frequent, vigorous exercise; and afterwards you should rub oil into your body. When you feel pangs of hunger, you may eat figs, as these are an excellent laxative.

We are bombarded daily, in magazines and on television, with dietary advice, some of which seem sensible, and some dubious. Hippocrates is the first dietary advisor in the western world whose words are still preserved; and he seems eminently sensible. And he raises two issues that are not normally mentioned today: the importance of modifying our diet according to the season; and the importance of not making major dietary changes during illness. The availability of all kinds of foods throughout the year means that most of us ignore the seasons; but our bodies are affected by the changing climate, and so it seems likely that our bodies need different foods in order to cope. Taking Hippocrates' advice as a starting point, would it be not be wise to make tentative alterations in our diet in summer, fall, winter and spring? As for times of illness, Hippocrates is expressing common sense, that this is not the time to put any additional strain on the body – and making major dietary changes is undoubtedly a strain.

CHAPTER 3

ENVIRONMENT

Consider first a district facing south, sheltered from cold, dry winds, but exposed to warm, humid breezes. If you live in such a place, you will have a moist head full of phlegm; this will flow down from the head and disturb your inner organs. Thus, if you are to avoid sickness, you will need to eat wisely and follow a strict routine.

Consider now a district facing north, sheltered from warm humid breezes, but exposed to cold, dry winds. If you live in such a place, you will tend to become lean and sturdy, prone to constipation but with a strong chest. You will have more trouble with bile than with phlegm; so you will suffer frequently from abscesses. You should ensure that you have ample food, but you should drink little wine.

Consider a district facing east, avoiding extremes of heat and cold. This is likely to provide the healthiest environment. If you live in such a place, you will have a good complexion, a loud and clear voice, and a robust temperament. You will suffer few diseases, and these will mainly be fevers that last only a short time.

Consider a district facing west, exposed to hot, moist winds in summer. If you live in such a place, the breezes will burn your skin, making your face rough and wrinkly, your voice will be thick and hoarse, and you will be prone to all manner of diseases. Again you will need to show special care over your diet, and you will need to exercise regularly.

From time to time medical experts analyze the incidence of different illnesses in different regions and countries; and it is striking how the figures vary. Heart disease, for example, is very common in some places, but quite rare in others; the same is true of some cancers and other life-threatening diseases, as well as many minor ailments. Sometimes there are obvious explanations, such as relative tobacco consumption or environmental pollution; but usually the experts can do no more than speculate. Hippocrates makes the simple point that the local climate is bound to affect the illnesses to which people are prone. And he asks us to reflect on our diet and our daily routine in relation to the local climate, in order to protect ourselves from the illnesses that are especially prevalent. Since each of us is different, and since every region has its own particular climate, he can give no general advice; but he indicates that, if we use of own intuition, we are likely to make the right judgments.

CHAPTER 4

WATER

Water plays a vital role in human health.

Stagnant water from marshes and lakes is warm and thick in the summer. In winter it is cold; and it is also muddy from rain running off the surrounding land. Such water tends to produce excessive phlegm, causing people to age rapidly die prematurely.

Water from rock springs is hard, containing various metals such as iron, copper, silver, gold or alum. This water is difficult to pass, and also tends to cause constipation.

The best water comes from springs high in the hills. It tends to be sweet and clean; and its temperature is even through the year, so it feels cool in summer and warm in winter.

If you enjoy good and robust health, you need not distinguish between one kind of water and another, but can drink whatever is at hand. But if your health is frail, or you are sick, then you must be careful, going to great lengths only to drink spring water.

The consumption of bottled water has grown enormously in recent decades, indicating that at last we have come to recognize – as Hippocrates recognized over two millennia ago – the importance of the quality of the water that we drink. But Hippocrates' advice may also help us to distinguish one kind of bottled water from another. We should prefer, especially during illness, water from mountain springs to water from mineral springs.

CHAPTER 5

BATHS, SLEEP AND MASSAGE

Regular bathing helps the body to resist illness. There should be no draughts in your bathroom, and you should use plenty of water. Do not rub yourself down with soap, but add a little soap to the water. Use a sponge rather than a scraper to clean the skin. Afterwards, while your skin is still wet, you should anoint yourself with oil. On no account should you let yourself become chilled, especially if you are sick. Do not bathe shortly after food or drink; and do not eat or drink shortly after a bath.

Sleep after a meal both aids digestion, and also enables the nourishment to spread across the body. Lack of sleep prevents the body receiving the nourishment from the food it has consumed. When you are sick, try to follow your normal pattern of sleep, spending the day awake and the night asleep. If you need more sleep is needed, take it in the late morning or early afternoon.

Massage warms the flesh and stimulates it. By compressing the flesh it draws nourishment to it. It also drives stale breath out of the body.

Many modern meals, particularly in the middle of the working day, are rushed, with no time to pause between mouthfuls, let alone relax afterwards. And at home many of us now graze, consuming food as we want, in the midst of other activities such as surfing the internet or watching television. Hippocrates invites us to reflect critically on this revolution in our eating habits. He also invites us to reflect on our bathing habits. Certainly we wash our bodies much more frequently than in the past; but many of us prefer the quick shower to the leisurely bath. None of us knows the long-term consequences on our physical and mental health of this hectic lifestyle; but, when we do reflect, we can only feel pessimistic – and consider how we might change.

CHAPTER 6

PAIN

As soon you feel any significant pain, you should rest; this will help to restore the bodily disturbances that cause the pain.

A pain in any part of the body is eased by the application of heat. Hot water should be put in a skin or bladder, or in an urn made of bronze or clay. A damp cloth or sponge should be put against the skin for comfort; and then the vessel of hot water placed on top. The hot vessel should itself be covered so that it remains hot longer.

If you have a pain in your head, you should warm your head by washing it in hot water. This may cause you to sneeze, which may further ease the pain. While the pain continues, you should not have a heavy meal, but should eat sparingly. And on no account should you drink wine until the pain has fully disappeared.

To ease pain in the back, boil celery and fennel bark in water, and then drink the water. Afterwards drink diluted white wine. Also wash the place where the pain is located in hot water; and then keep a warm poultice on the place.

There are numerous analgesics on the market, and most of us have packets of pain-killing pills in a bedroom drawer, to take when headache or backache strikes. But Hippocrates suggests methods, especially the application of heat, that ease both the pain and its causes. The modern electrically heated pad seems a reasonable substitute for Hippocrates' urn of bronze and clay.

CHAPTER 7

COMMON AILMENTS

Catarrh. If after a common cold the nose remains congested, and the complexion remains pallid, action should be taken; letting matters drift can cause considerable damage. When you are at rest the mucus becomes thicker and the nasal passages more congested - which is why the problem is greatest after dinner or after sleep. But when you are warmed by exercise, the mucus thins, and the nose becomes less congested. Thus you should take more vigorous exercise, not to the point of becoming fatigued, but in order to warm thoroughly the whole body. Each act of vigorous exercise should be followed by a warm bath. You should also flush out the mouth and throat at least once a day with a harsh, astringent wine - being careful not to swallow any.

Diarrhea. This can cause great weakness, because it prevents the stomach from deriving nutrition from the food that you eat. The treatment is to fast, eating nothing, so that the digestive system can relax completely. No wine should be taken; but you may drink the juice of white grapes to quench your thirst. You may also drink the juice obtained when lentils or beans are cooked.

Wounds. When the skin has been cut, and especially if the wound has been inflamed, apply a plaster made from beet, celery, olive leaves, fig leaves or sweet pomegranate. The plaster should first be boiled. Under no circumstances should fat be applied to a wound, as this will worsen the inflammation. However, once the wound has begun to heal, fat or oil may be rubbed gently into the new tissue, to aid its growth.

Sciatica and arthritis. Sciatica is greatly eased by warm baths, and by applying heat to the area of pain. Arthritis is eased by cold baths, and by applying coolness to the joints that cause pain. Drinking boiled milk can also help.

Hiccups. Drink vinegar and honey. Boil the vinegar and honey separately, and then mix them. This may be supplemented by a gruel made with barley, to which a little honey has been added. And if hiccups persist, strong white wine should be taken.

If Hippocrates came back to life today, he would not stick dogmatically to the remedies he prescribed in ancient times. Nor would he forbid the use of modern drugs. But, as his first principles state, he would urge us first to use simple remedies that enhance the body's own powers of healing. If these fail, then we can turn to medicines that rely on their own powers. As for which simple remedies we should try, he would advise us to learn from one another's experience; and happily today there are numerous books and articles in which simple remedies are suggested for different ailments.

CHAPTER 8

DREAMS

When your dreams are simply a continuation of your daytime actions and thoughts, this indicates that your body and soul are healthy. But when your dreams involve conflict and violence, your body and soul are disturbed; and the degree of conflict and violence indicates the seriousness of the disturbances.

As soon as you became aware of violent dreams, you should have only a light diet for at least five days, you should have a brisk walk early in the morning, and you should do vigorous exercises in the gym; you should also exercise your voice. All this will help calm the disturbance.

If, however, the violent dreams continue, you should have long runs, wearing heavy clothes, so the body sweats profusely. You should also have no breakfast, and reduce your other meals even further. Moreover, you should replace normal foods with foods that are dry, pungent and bitter.

There are various indications in dreams that your body and soul are returning to health. These include seeing clearly and hearing distinctly, walking firmly without stumbling, and running swiftly. Also the earth in your dreams will appear smooth and well-tilled, the trees will have bright, green leaves and be laden with fruit, rivers will flow easily with abundant clear water, and the sun will shine brightly.

Specific ailments can be discerned through images in dreams.

If you dream of eating your normal food, this indicates undernourishment. If a particular food seems to have a strong taste, this indicates that you are deficient in that food. If you dream of fleeing from something, this indicates you are dehydrated, and should drink more.

If you dream of being attacked by enemy soldiers, this indicates the onset of madness – for which the best antidote is vigorous exercise, a diet of soft food, frequent warm baths, and ample rest.

If in your dreams you cannot see or hear properly, this indicates some illness in the head; longer walks in the early morning and after dinner will usually cure the problem.

If you see trees that are losing their leaves, the cause is excessive coldness and moisture in your body; so you must have extra heating in your home, and drink less. If you see trees that are barren, this indicates excessive heat and lack of moisture in your body – so you have less heat in your home, and drink more.

If in a dream a river is not flowing normally, this indicates problems with your blood. If the amount of water is greater than normal, there is superfluity of blood; if it is less, there is deficiency. If the water is cloudy, there is disturbance in the smooth flow of blood. In each case the cause is insufficient air coming into the body; you must learn to breathe more deeply.

If you see a spring not flowing properly, this indicates problems with your bladder passing water; you should take a diuretic. If you encounter a rough sea in a dream, this indicates problems in the bowels, causing constipation; you should take a laxative.

If you are sick, an earth tremor or the shaking of a house in a dream predicts that you will soon recover – so you should begin to eat and exercise more. If you are well, the same images predict that you will soon fall ill so you should reduce your food and exercise.

If you see a land flooded with water, or you dream of diving into water, you have excess fluid in the body; so you should drink less and eat drier foods. If you see land that is black and scorched, your body is dehydrated; so you should drink more and eat moist foods. Stop exercise, and do not eat dry, pungent diuretic food. Instead have boiled barley water and small quantities of light food, together with plenty of diluted white wine; and take frequent baths.

Freud pioneered the interpretation of dreams as a means of uncovering our unconscious urges; but, since unconscious urges can never be known directly, it has been impossible to test whether such interpretations are correct. There is also a long tradition of interpreting dreams as omens. But Hippocrates suggests another use of dreams, which has had remarkably little attention: the early diagnosis of illnesses, and thence the indication of appropriate remedies. And since illnesses can be directly known, it is possible to test the validity of his interpretations, and to develop additional interpretations along similar lines. Indeed, we can each try it for ourselves. If Hippocrates is right, this could prove a hugely powerful weapon in the medical armory – which, unlike most other weapons, costs absolutely nothing.

Pliny

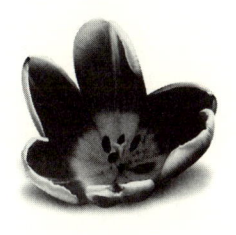

Plants as Medicines

INTRODUCTION

Pliny's *Natural History* is an encyclopedia of scientific knowledge amongst the Romans in the first century CE. One part of it concerns the science of health and medicine; and in particular he describes the healing powers of various plants.

Pliny was born in 23 CE northern Italy, and began his career in the army, serving mainly in Germany. He then held administrative positions in Gaul, Africa and Spain. He returned to Rome in 75, and spent the last four years of his life writing.

CHAPTER I

SYMPATHY AND ANTIPATHY

None of us fully realizes the degree to which health is maintained and restored by particular plants. The names of these plants are so mundane that they give no hint of their wonderful qualities.

When we look at Nature, we see that she is sometimes at peace with herself, and sometimes in conflict. The same applies to plants in relation to us: some plants are at peace with us, and some in conflict. We may call plants at peace with us 'sympathetic', and plants in conflict with us 'antipathetic'.

There is increasing evidence of animals using plants to treat their own illnesses – chimpanzees eating certain leaves to cure stomach upsets, elephants eating fermented berries to overcome stress, and so on. Equally animals are very adept at avoiding plants that might do them harm. So if animals can distinguish between sympathetic and antipathetic plants, should we not do the same? Then, as Pliny suggests, we can act to a great extent as our own physicans.

CHAPTER 2

VEGETABLES

Cabbage. **Raw cabbage, especially the varieties with curly leaves,** relieves headaches, improves eyesight, and reduces anxiety. Steamed cabbage, when it is placed on wounds, stops bleeding and promotes healing. Streamed cabbage, when eaten at the evening meal, prevents both insomnia and unpleasant dreams. Chronic insomniacs should eat only steamed cabbage with oil and salt in the evening.

Cucumber. The seeds of cucumbers improve poor eyesight, and heal diseases on the eyes and eyelids. The seeds are crushed and put in rainwater, where they sink to the bottom. The mixture is left in the sun until the water has evaporated. The remaining substance is smeared on the eyelids and the eyes. The roots of cucumbers heal impetigo, scabies, psoriasis and ringworm. The roots are dried and compounded with resin, and then smeared on the infected area.

Lettuce. This helps to induce sleep, cools a feverish body, purges the stomach, disperse flatulence, and restrains sexual desire. It also balances the appetite: if people are inclined to eat too much, lettuce checks their appetite; if they tend to eat too little, lettuce stimulates it. Excessive amounts of lettuce can cause diarrhea.

Onion. The smell of onions brings tears to the eyes; and this helps poor eyesight. It is even more effective to apply onion juice directly to the eyes. Raw onions eaten with bread heal mouth ulcers; and raw onions eaten at bedtime help to induce sleep. Some say that eating onions promotes a healthy complexion, and that onions used as a suppository cure hemorrhoids.

CHAPTER 3

FLOWERS AND HERBS

Helenium. This enhances the complexion, especially of women. Its aroma stimulates sexual desire in men; so it may be made into a perfume for women.

Garlic. This is very helpful when people move from place to another. As they drink different water and breathe different air, their internal organs are disturbed, leading to all kinds of ailments. Garlic helps the internal organs to adapt, and so prevents those ailments.

Pennyroyal. The aroma of pennyroyal relieves headaches, and helps to prevent colds and fevers; so a garland of it should be placed in the bedroom. People working in the sun are less likely to suffer heat stroke if they have sprigs of pennyroyal behind their ears. When it is boiled with honey and soda, and drunk, pennyroyal cures disorders of the intestines; and taken in wine it helps to disperse stones in the kidney.

Poppy. Poppy seeds, pounded into tablets and added to milk, relieve pain and induce sleep. When people have an incurable disease causing acute pain, they yearn to die; a large dose of poppy seed tablets brings a peaceful death.

Thyme. This herb flowers at about the time of the summer solstice; and this is when the bees collect from it. Honey from thyme flowers is the most potent of all medicines, and is effective against almost all illnesses.

CHAPTER 4

GRAPE JUICES

Vinegar. This is noted both for its cooling properties, and also for its capacity to cause things to disintegrate. Inhaling vinegar checks nausea, hiccups, coughs and sneezes; it also relieves catarrh. Holding vinegar in the mouth brings down a fever. People convalescing from illness should gargle vinegar, as this increases their energy and helps them to digest food. Vinegar is also an antidote to insect and snakebites. But it should only be used as a seasoning in very small quantities, as it harms the bladder.

Wine taken in moderate quantities increases a person's resistance to disease, and also helps to maintain a happy, cheerful disposition. But taken in excessive quantities it has the opposite effects.

CHAPTER 5

TREES

Holly. A mixture of crushed holly leaves and salt can be rubbed on joints to relieve pain and stiffness. Holly berries are good for stomach disorders, dysentery and cholera; and taken in wine they cure diarrhea. Boiled holly root, when applied to the skin, reduces swellings.

Ivy. Juice from the ivy, when dropped into the nose, clears the head; it is even more effective when mixed with soda. It may also be dropped into the ear to relieve earache.

Juniper. Berries from the juniper tree relieve toothache: when they are chewed, they cause the aching tooth to break and fall out. Juice from the berries is sometimes recommended for indigestion; drops of the juice in the ear help to cure deafness; and smeared on the penis before sexual intercourse the juice is an effective contraceptive. But it is extremely powerful, and should only be used very sparingly.

Oak. Ground acorns, compounded wit salt and axle-grease, should be smeared onto calluses. Acorns boiled in water are helpful for stomach disorders and dysentery. The shell should always be left on the acorn, since the shell and the underlying pith are the most potent parts.
Terebinth. Resin dissolved in oil cleanses and closes up wounds. Also smeared on the chest it cures chest ailments. When it is warmed, it may be rubbed on limbs to relieve pains in the muscles and joints.

Walnut. Each part of the walnut tree has medicinal uses. Fresh walnuts, consumed in large quantities, expel tapeworms. Old walnuts cure gangrene, carbuncles and bruises. The bark of walnut trees cures ringworm and dysentery. And pounded walnut leaves mixed with vinegar cure earache.

Pliny's work is a compendium of the medical wisdom of his time as it related to plants. Thus he describes remedies that had been developed and used over centuries. This does not mean that they are all effective: people can cling on to all kinds of false notions for a long time. Nonetheless there is a slow process of natural selection in popular medical remedies: if a remedy consistently fails, then it is likely to be used less and less often, until it is finally forgotten; while if a remedy frequently succeeds, it will be used more and more often. Yet this process has gone through a strange kind of revolution in modern western society. On the one hand, pharmaceutical companies have been using this traditional wisdom to develop new drugs, which they then test in a systematic manner; so the rejection of ineffective remedies, and the acceptance of effective ones, has been greatly hastened. On the other hand, the ready availability of pharmaceutical drugs means that we are quickly forgetting the traditional remedies that had been handed down the generations; so soon there will be no traditional wisdom left. Should we deliberately attempt to revive the kind of remedies that Pliny describes, and then hand them on to our children? Are we prepared to go to the extra trouble of using traditional remedies, instead of merely buying drugs in packets? The main practical case for reviving traditional remedies is that, even if their benign effects are slow or even negligible, they are unlikely to have any malign side effects.

Raja Yoga

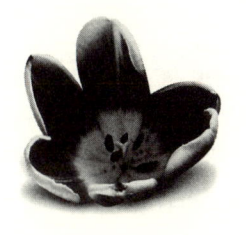

DISCIPLINE OF THE MIND

INTRODUCTION

Yoga means 'discipline', and *raja* means 'royal'. When the two words are brought together as a single term, *Raja Yoga*, it is usually understood as 'discipline of the mind'. Its purpose is to overcome all kinds of anxiety, depression and stress, and thence bring contentment and serenity.

The techniques of Raja Yoga were probably developed thousands of years ago by the sages of northern India; and undoubtedly by the time the major Hindu scriptures were compiled in the first millennium BCE, they were widely practiced. In c4 a man called Patanjali set them down in the form of a manual by a man; and over the centuries this manual, called the *Yoga Sutra*, became hugely popular.

Nothing is known about Patanjali, but it is reasonable to suppose that he followed the normal pattern of life of a Hindu *sannyasin*. As a young man he would have left his family, and spent several years as the disciple of a *guru*. Then he may have lived alone in a hut or a cave, gradually accumulating disciples of his own; or he may have wandered from place to place, teaching people whom he encountered.

The central element of Raja Yoga is meditation, in which the mind fixes itself on a particular object or sound; and through regular meditation the mind gradually becomes free of all disturbance, and attains a state of superior consciousness. In order to practice meditation successfully, the posture must be both firm and relaxed, and breathing should be deep and steady. Similar techniques can be found in all the major religions of the world; but Patanjali's work has pride of place for the clarity and simplicity of his exposition.

CHAPTER I

FREEDOM FROM DISTURBANCES

Yoga is concerned with freedom from mental disturbances. Through Yoga the soul becomes perfectly serene; and without Yoga the soul is in constant turmoil.

There are five kinds of disturbance: observation; doubt; idealism; pessimism; and memory. By observation we mean perceiving external objects, drawing inferences about them, and learning about them from others. By doubt we mean concern about the possibility that something may be different from what it appears. By idealism we mean the external goals or ambitions that we set ourselves. By pessimism we mean an outlook that regards evil as genuine. By memory we mean attributing to external objects continuing and indefinite reality.

To become free from mental disturbances requires effort and patience. By effort we mean persistent attempts to attain serenity; and persistence implies constant and uninterrupted devotion. By patience we mean willingness gradually to relinquish all attachment to external objects, both seen and heard; this willingness implies an acceptance of one's fate, whatever it may be.

None of us is free from mental disturbances; almost all of us go through periods of considerable mental turmoil; and some of us lead lives that are blighted by mental problems of one kind or another. Oddly, however, many of us make no serious attempt to address our inner difficulties; we delude ourselves that outward things – affluence, career success, and so on – will bring us happiness. Patanjali, gently and without moral pressure, invites us to abandon this delusion, and to look inwards.

CHAPTER 2

SUPERIOR CONSCIOUSNESS

Normal consciousness is concerned with reasoning, distinguishing one object from another, enjoyment and self-awareness. There is also superior consciousness, in which all mental activity ceases; this attained through various stages.

Some have a natural tendency towards superior consciousness, which they have inherited from their forbears. Others must attain superior consciousness through strong conviction, intense effort, deep study, firm concentration, and profound spiritual discernment.

Those who wish to attain superior consciousness should seek and emulate an ideal soul. An ideal soul is one who is unmoved by physical temptations, by promises of reward, and by bodily cravings.

In the ideal soul knowledge is at its highest level. And the symbol of the ideal soul is the sound *Aum*. Repetition of *Aum*, and understanding of its significance, helps towards the attainment of superior consciousness.

Is superior consciousness something utterly distinct from normal consciousness? Does the human mind have the potential for another type of consciousness, besides the consciousness that all human minds experience? Or is superior consciousness a development of normal consciousness? The mind is undoubtedly capable of different states of consciousness: the state of consciousness during dreaming is quite different from waking consciousness. Patanjali is suggesting a third state of consciousness; but unlike dreaming, which is involuntary, superior consciousness is attained by deliberate effort. The real question that Patanjali is putting to us is this: are we really motivated to make this effort?

CHAPTER 3

STAGES OF MEDITATION

In order to attain superior consciousness, you must learn to meditate, which means transcending the relationship between perception and the objects of perception. This has three stages.

The first stage is steadying the mind. Concentrating on a plant, or a light, of an inanimate object, steadies the mind. Some find it easiest to hold the mind steady when they are in a dreamy or sleepy state. The method of steadying the mind is a matter of personal choice.

Once a steady mind has been attained, it is time to consider the relationship between the perceiver and the objects perceived. This relationship is concerned with the words used to describe the objects, the inferences that are drawn about objects, the distinctions made between one object and another, and doubts about the nature of the objects. All these issues disturb the mind. So the second stage is to exclude them from consciousness.

The third stage is freedom from desire for objects. Only when consciousness is freed from all desire does the true nature of things become clear; free from desire, the mind sees through the veil of appearance, and becomes aware of reality. Ordinary knowledge, obtained through observation and inference, sees only particular truths about things; the mind free from desire must not even desire the awareness that such freedom brings. Freedom from desire yields true enjoyment in the mind.

Through most of the day our minds flit from one thing to another; but then occasionally they settle and become steady. In order to meditate, we must learn to steady our minds at will; and this is largely a matter of practice. Through most of the day the thoughts within our minds form a kind of film, with ourselves as spectators. Patanjali is telling us to stop the film, and let the screen go blank. Like a real film, our thoughts evoke feelings, both positive and negative. Patanjali is telling us that, when our mental screen goes blank, we must also let our feelings subside. All this sounds very dull: who wants to sit in front of a blank screen, feeling nothing? Yet Patanjali assures us – and everyone experienced in meditation can confirm this – that a deeper enjoyment takes the place of normal desires and pleasures; and this enjoyment is lasting, and is free from pain.

CHAPTER 4

HINDRANCES TO MEDITATION

There are five hindrances to successful meditation: ignorance, egoism, attachment, aversion, and tenacity. Ignorance is the soil in which the other hindrances grow; it consists in mistaking the transient for the eternal, the impure for the pure, evil for good, the apparent self for the real self. Egoism consists in identifying the soul, which is the source of awareness, with the instruments of awareness, which are the senses and the mind. Attachment consists in being tied to the causes of pleasure. Aversion consists in being fearful of the causes of pain. Tenacity consists in clinging to bodily life.

These five hindrances can gradually be overcome by persistent effort; and this effort can only be properly directed if you recognize the hindrances within yourself. Every thought and action either strengthens or weakens the hindrances.

So long as the hindrances remain, they determine your roles in life, the length of your life, and the joys and sorrows you experience through life. Joy is the fruit of thoughts and actions that weaken hindrances; and sorrow is the fruit of thoughts and actions that strengthen hindrances. Yet even at moments of joy there will always be inner turmoil, until full superior consciousness has been attained.

Overcoming the hindrances to meditation is where the greatest effort is required; and this effort must be sustained through every hour of every day. Whenever we are asserting ourselves over others; whenever we are trying to further our own personal interests; whenever we are setting out to the shopping mall in order to buy some new object that we desire; whenever we are relishing our own status or power – we must stop ourselves and reflect. Is any good purpose served by our self-assertion? What are our genuine interests, and are they perhaps identical with other people's? Will that new object really bring any additional happiness? And what's so great about status and power? Patanjali is asking us to ask ourselves these types of questions constantly. And when we ask then, they virtually answer themselves. After a while the questions become so habitual that we barely need to articulate them; that is the sign that we are beginning to win the battle.

CHAPTER 5

ASPECTS OF MEDITATION

There are five external aspects of meditation: abstinence, devotion, right posture, right breathing, and retracting the senses.

Abstinence consists in abstaining from five things: injuring other people or any other living beings; speaking dishonestly and giving false impressions; taking things that belong to other people or any other living beings; becoming attached to particular pleasures and their causes; becoming attached to particular external objects. These abstinences are universal, and must be practiced in all places, times and circumstances, and in every aspect of your life.

Devotion consists in being devoted to five things: cleanliness, both inward and outward; serenity; self-control; self-knowledge; and to the ideal of superior consciousness. Abstinence and devotion go together, since abstinence from that which is evil implies devotion to that which is good.

The right posture is firm and comfortable. Right posture comes from reducing the tendency towards restlessness; and restlessness of the body arises from tensions in the mind. These tensions must be eased. Right breathing depends on controlling the motions of inhaling and exhaling. You are breathing badly if your inhalations are too shallow, and your exhalations too rapid. When you are breathing badly, your mind is constantly being disturbed. When you breathe easily and freely, your mind becomes more peaceful, and you are better able to concentrate the mind.

Retracting the senses means paying no more attention to objects of pleasure than to any other objects. This requires complete control of the senses.

The physical requirements for successful meditation are, according to Patanjali, quite simple: a comfortable posture in which the body is fully relaxed; and calm, steady breathing. The moral requirements, however, are much more demanding. In Patanjali's scheme, meditation is not purely a technique to improve our state of mind and make us happier; it is closely connected with the way in which we treat other people and other living beings. If we cause harm, then we cannot successful meditate; and uttering any kind of falsehood will also thwart our efforts. And the avoidance of causing harm requires constant vigilance, since injury through carelessness is just as bad as deliberate injury. So before we even begin to learn meditation, we must ask ourselves whether we are willing to practice such tight moral discipline.

CHAPTER 6

SIGNS OF SUPERIOR CONSCIOUSNESS

In a state of superior consciousness the mind is unconscious of itself. As a result all mental disturbance ceases, and the mind experiences harmony within itself. Moreover, the mind no longer regards itself as a distinct entity, and hence it ceases to make a distinction between harmony and disturbance. The mind knows itself and the body perfectly; yet it does not know itself or the body at all.

In a state of superior consciousness the mind ceases to distinguish between past and future; they are perceived as one. The mind ceases to use words to distinguish between entities, because all things are perceived as one. thus words have lost their meaning.

In a state of superior consciousness the mind is able to apprehend the thoughts of other minds; it can perceive clearly the attachments that disturb other minds. The five senses are heightened and clarified, because the mind is not disturbed by what the senses perceive. The distinction between actions that are intended, and those that are unintended, disappears, since the mind can always anticipate the effects of the actions that it prompts.

In a state of superior consciousness the mind is consistently friendly towards other people, and it has no wish to exercise power over others.

In a state of superior consciousness the mind ceases to use logic as a means of understanding; intuition is sufficient. The mind is not swayed by emotion, nor does it control the emotions; mind and heart are perfectly unified. The mind is free from slavery to the body, so bodily hunger and thirst cannot disturb it, sound and silence become one.

In a state of superior consciousness the mind no longer perceives time as a line, in which one moment follows another; and it no longer perceives space as separating one thing from another.

Occasionally we encounter people who are not only very serene and tranquil, but also seem to have a profound and immediate understanding of others; we feel they see right into us. Sometimes such people become hailed as great spiritual leaders; but they themselves prefer to live in obscurity, and many do – so we may meet them in quite ordinary circumstances. According to Patanjali's terminology, they have attained superior consciousness. And although they may not have followed Patanjali's instructions, they will have followed the path he describes, since this path, with minor variations, is taught in all spiritual traditions. Yet there is a strange paradox about such people, to which Patanjali alludes: while they are deeply aware of others, and while they have mastered their own thoughts and feelings, they are not in the least self-conscious. Indeed, they no longer think of themselves as distinct selves. Do we seriously wish to lose all sense of self? If we can answer that positively, then we can begin to go down Patanjali's path. But if our answer is negative, we should turn away.

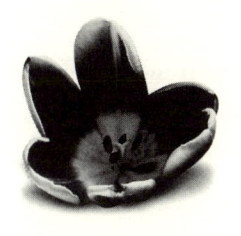

Hatha Yoga

DISCIPLINE OF THE BODY

INTRODUCTION

Hatha means 'physical exertion'. Thus *Hatha Yoga* is the discipline of the body through exertion. Its purpose is to prevent and cure illnesses of every kind, and to enhance people's energy so that they remain vigorous and youthful.

Hatha Yoga seems to have emerged in India in c9 CE. The first exponent was called Matsyendranath, and he acquired a large group of disciples. Gradually its techniques spread through the general population of India; and while some its more extreme practices were confined to only a few stalwarts, its basic forms were widely adopted. Then in c19 visitors from western countries discovered it; and now people throughout the world include Hatha Yoga as part of a healthy way of life.

A teacher called Svatmarama wrote the classic exposition of Hatha Yoga in c15. In a series of clear, short verses he outlines its three main aspects. The first is a series of postures, each of which brings specific physical benefits. The second is a program of breathing exercises. The third consists of various means of cleansing the inner organs of the body. He also offers some simple advice about diet.

CHAPTER 1

CONDITIONS FOR YOGA

There are conflicting religious doctrines; but these doctrines merely darken the mind, and so prevent people from attaining wisdom through the mind. Yet wisdom can be found also through the body.

Yoga of the body can quench the fires of suffering that consume the mind and the body.

If you wish to acquire supernatural powers, you must practice yoga in secret. If you reveal your practice of yoga to others without discrimination, your efforts will be in vain.

You should practice yoga in a place where you are alone and free from disturbance. You may create for yourself a hermitage. It should have a small door; and it should have no windows, so you can neither be seen nor distracted.

Sitting in such a place you should free your mind from all stray thoughts. Then you are ready to practice yoga.

The energy necessary for yoga is dissipated by excessive eating and by excessive fasting, by heavy manual labor and by physical idleness, by sexual abstinence and by promiscuous sexual activity.

Success in yoga of the body depends on being cheerful; on perseverance and courage; on being aware of yourself; and on the avoidance of unnecessary social activity.

Success also depends on not causing suffering to any living being; on speaking the truth; on not taking what belongs to others; on being sexually faithful to your spouse; on showing compassion and kindness to others; on being quick to forgive the wrong that others do to you; and on being moderate in your diet.

If Hatha Yoga is practiced merely as a program of physical exercises, it undoubtedly yields physical benefits. But it will not lead to wholeness of mind and body – it will not bring genuine good health. It must be aligned, according to Svatmarama, with a high degree of mental and moral discipline, of the kind advocated by Patanjali; so Hatha Yoga and Raja Yoga are complementary, not competing, techniques. Some people, however, undertake Hatha Yoga purely for its spiritual benefits, imagining that if they master its complex postures, they will become holy, and may even acquire supernatural powers. Svatmarama tells us that this motivation leads to two peculiar paradoxes. First, while Hatha Yoga may indeed help to make us holy, we cannot acquire holiness by wanting it for its own sake; on the contrary, desiring holiness for ourselves prevents us from acquiring it. Secondly, while Hatha Yoga may indeed give us supernatural powers, we can only successfully practice Hatha Yoga by setting aside all doctrines and beliefs about the supernatural.

CHAPTER 2

POSTURES

Sit cross-legged on the ground, and squeeze each foot between the calf and the thigh of the opposite leg.

Place the right foot next to the left buttock, and the left foot next to the right buttock. This posture looks like the mouth of a cow.

Place one foot upon the opposite thigh, and the other foot beneath the opposite thigh.

Kneel down, and cross your feet; then sit on your crossed feet – but do so with care.

Sit cross-legged, with each foot placed on the opposite thigh, tucked as close to the body as possible. This is the lotus posture.

In the lotus posture insert your hands between your calves and your thighs. Put your palms firmly on the ground, and push so that you raise your body from the ground.

Sitting on the ground, grasp the big toe of your left foot with your left hand, and the big tow of your right foot with your left hand. Keep the left leg straight and pull the right foot to your ear. Then keep the right leg straight and pull the left foot to your ear.

Sitting on the ground, tuck your right foot into your left buttock, and put your left leg over your right knee so that the foot is on the ground.

Grasp the left foot with the right hand, passing the arm to the left side of the knee; and turn your head as far as possible to the left. Undertake the same posture the other way round. This increases the appetite by fanning the gastric fires, and thereby heals those illnesses caused by the gastric fires burning too weakly.

Sitting on the ground, stretch out your legs, and lean forward until you can grasp your toes; as you do so, rest your head on your knees. This helps your breath to flow freely, energizes the spinal column, increases the appetite, makes the hip supple, and heals those illness causes by lack of vigor.

Lie face down. Press your palms firmly on the ground, and raise yourself, balancing your body by pressing the elbows on the hips. Stretch your legs outwards so that your feet are level with your head. This posture heals the various diseases of the spleen, it causes swellings to subside, and it helps your digestion when you have eaten excessively.

Lie on your back like a corpse. This eliminates the tiredness caused by other postures, and also relieves mental stress.

Sit cross-legged, with the left foot pressed into the body below the sex organs, and the right foot resting on the left calf; or you may sit with your legs and feet the opposite way round. Pull your body upright, so that your spinal column is straight and your chin pressed back. This posture is good for meditation. If you perform it regularly, and control your breathing carefully, then in twelve years you will attain utter tranquility.

Sitting on the ground, place the right foot at the top of the left thigh, and place the left foot at the top of the right thigh. Crossing your arms behind your back, grasp the big toe of your right foot with your right hand, and the big toe of your left foot with your left hand. Bow your head, resting your chin on your chest. This helps to cure every kind of disease.

Sitting in the lotus posture, curl your tongue backwards so that it touches the upper teeth at the back of your mouth. Rest your chin on your chest, and breathe slowly, while clasping your hands tightly together. This too helps the cure every kind of disease.

In this posture, meditate on divinity, frequently clenching your buttocks and swallowing hard. This helps to liberate the mind.

Sitting on the ground with your body upright, pull your foot under your buttocks, your left foot under your left buttock, and your right foot under your right buttock. This helps to relieve any pain.

Some people are born supple, and so can accomplish the yoga postures with relative ease; while others with naturally stiff joints have great difficulty. And all of us grow stiffer with age. This seems to suggest that only the young and supple should undertake Hatha Yoga. This is partly true: the yoga postures lie at the heart of Hatha Yoga; and if they are utterly impossible, there is no point in trying. Yet it is important to maintain as much suppleness as age and nature allow: this not only promotes physical health, but also aids relaxation, which is a vital component of meditation. And a gentle form of Hatha Yoga, gradually learning to accomplish some of the simpler postures, is one means of doing this.

CHAPTER 3

DIET

You should always stop eating when you are still a little hungry. Leave a quarter of your stomach empty.

You should avoid foods that are sour, pungent or spicy. These include mustard, alcoholic drinks, fish, meat, curds, buttermilk, chickpeas, linseed cake, and garlic.

You should never reheat your food.

You should avoid foods that are excessively salty or acidic, and also foods that woody and hard to chew.

You can eat these foods without hesitation: wheat products such as bread; rice, milk, honey, dried ginger, cucumbers, and vegetables of all kinds. You may also drink as much fresh water as you wish.

You can practice yoga at any age and in any state. You may be young, old, or even very old. You may be strong or frail. You may be healthy or sickly. Yoga helps people in all conditions.

It is no good cramming yoga sessions into a hectic lifestyle, in which meals consist of junk food consumed at speed. Svatmarama tells us that, if we wish to practice Hatha Yoga successfully, we must eat healthily, consuming simple, nutritious food in the right quantities. Svatmarama, of course, lived long before it was possible to measure and count calories. But he offers a simple way of avoiding excessive consumption: we should rise from meals before our hunger is fully satisfied. This has the added benefit of instilling self-control, so that we become masters, instead of slaves, of our desires.

CHAPTER 4

BREATHING EXERCISES

When the breath is unsteady, so also is the mind. When the breath is calm and tranquil, the mind also is calm and tranquil. Therefore you should learn to control your breath.

Breathing cleanses and purifies the channels within the body. If these channels are clogged with impurities, the body becomes sick. So by breathing well you can make yourself well.

Sit on the ground, preferably in the lotus posture. Close your right nostril, and inhale through your left nostril. Hold your breath. Then close your left nostril, and exhale through your right nostril. Now close your left nostril, and inhale through your right nostril. Hold your breath. Then close your right nostril, and exhale through your left nostril. Do this many times, so that you are always inhaling through the same nostril from which you have just exhaled.

In this breathing exercise you should hold your breath either until your skin starts to perspire, or your whole body starts to tremble. Do not then exhale suddenly and rapidly, but exhale slowly and gradually. In this way your body gains greater and greater energy.

You should practice this breathing exercise four times a day: early in the morning soon after you rise; at midday; at dusk; and shortly before you retire for the night. Gradually increase the time you spend, until can perform eighty rounds – inhaling through your left nostril eighty times, and through your right nostril eighty times.

Through practice you will find that you can hold your breath for longer and longer before your skin perspires or your body trembles.

When you have finished your breathing exercise, massage your body. This gives you agility and strength.

During the rest of the day you will find that you breathe more deeply and calmly, and so your mind is calmer.

If you breathe badly, you will tend to suffer from cough, asthma, headaches, and pain in the eyes and ears. If you learn to breathe well, these illnesses will be cured.

Becoming aware of breathing, and learning to control it, is central to all guidance on meditation; and Svatmarama's advice can be found in countless other books. But Svatmarama emphasizes a point that is often lost: that we should concentrate not on the chest, lungs and diaphragm which are the sources of breathing, but on the nostrils through which breath is inhaled and exhaled. If we try to focus on our inner organs, we quickly feel tense, because we cannot properly be aware of them, and hence cannot directly control them. But we are fully aware of our nostrils; and we control breath by focusing on them.

CHAPTER 5

CLEANSING THE BODY

There are six methods of cleansing the body. These have numerous wonderful results, and so they are highly valued amongst those who practice yoga.

The first method is this. Take a strip of clean cloth, which is about four fingers wide and fifteen fingers long. Slowly swallow it. Then pull it back out. This is a remedy for asthma, illness of the pancreas, and leprosy.

The second method is this. Crouch in a tub of water, with your heels pressed against your buttocks. The water should come as high as your navel. Insert a bamboo pipe into the anus, and contract the anus to draw in water. This is a remedy for illness of the spleen, and for constipation. It helps the bodily fluids to flow more smoothly, enhances the senses, and strengthens the heart. It also makes the skin glow, and increases the appetite.

The third method is this. Pull a thread, four fingers in length, through one of the nostrils, and let it emerge through the mouth. This cleanses the head, and makes the eyes sharp. It also heals any illness of the neck and head. The fourth method is this. Gaze without blinking on some small object until tears come into your eyes. This cures any illness in the eyes, and also overcomes fatigue.

The fifth method is this. Bend your head forward, and slowly rotate your belly like a whirlpool in a river. This stimulates the digestion, and helps the entire body to relax.

The sixth method is this. Inhale and exhale rapidly and deeply, like the bellows of a blacksmith. This strengthens the body's resistance to disease.

Only a few yoga practitioners have ever used the first four of Svatmarama's cleansing exercises – although the second practice bears some resemblance to colonic irrigation, a therapy that has gained popularity in recent years. Each of them has obvious and serious dangers. The fifth practice is perfectly safe, and some people find it quite easy.

CHAPTER 6

USING THE BREATH

There are eight ways of using the breath.

The first way is this. Inhale deeply, and hold your breath. Press your chin against your chest, and pull your belly inwards. When you can hold your breath no longer, lift your head straight, release your belly, and exhale as fully as possible.

The second way is this. Inhale deeply, and hold your breath. Clench your buttocks tightly. This will force the air through the inner channels of your body.

The third way is this. Inhale deeply through the right nostril, and hold your breath for as long as possible. Then exhale as fully as possible. Now do the same, inhaling through your left nostril. Repeat this several times until your whole body, from your head to your toes, is suffused with breath. This cleanses the brain and the sinuses, destroys intestinal worms, and cures flatulence.

The fourth way is this. Close your mouth and inhale through your nostrils as deeply as you can, so that breath fills your lungs completely. The last part of this inhalation causes a whistling noise; this shows that the tips of your lungs are being filled. Now exhale through the left nostril. Do the same, exhaling through the right nostril. This removes the phlegm in your throat, and helps the digestion. It may be practiced either sitting or walking.

The fifth way is this. Push your tongue a little way through your lips. Then inhale through the mouth, making a hissing sound, hold your breath, and exhale through the nostrils. Repeat this many times. It makes the skin shine, controls hunger and thirst, overcomes fatigue, and enhances muscular strength.

The sixth way is this. Push your tongue as far out as it will go. Then inhale through the mouth, making a hissing sound, hold your breath, and exhale through the nostrils. Repeat this many times. It overcomes fever, relieves pain in the gall bladder, helps to overcome hunger and thirst, and renders harmless the poison from snakebites.

The seventh way is this. Exhale through the nostrils, keeping you mouth closed; and continue exhaling, pushing the air from your lungs, until you can feel pressure on your heart, throat and head. Then inhale deeply through your mouth; but only open your mouth a little, so the air makes a hissing sound as it enters. Keep you neck and body straight throughout this exercise. This saturates your body with breath.

The eighth way is this. Inhale rapidly, making the sound a male bee, and exhale slowly, making the sound of a female bee. This brings great emotional tranquility and joy.

These eight ways, when they are followed regularly, make the body more agile and the mind more nimble, and they increase sexual potency.

It would be almost impossible to prove that any of the exercises recommended by Svatmarama have the particular benefits he ascribes to them. But does this mean that undertaking these exercises is a matter of blind faith? Indeed, this same question can be applied to all health practices that do not involve modern drugs – especially those that are quite time-consuming. How can we decide whether a particular practice is worthwhile, when no formal scientific tests have been done on its efficacy? The fact is that such tests are very expensive; and generally only the international drug companies have the financial resources – and the legal requirement – to perform them. Tradition is a kind of informal test. If a practice stands the test of time – decades, centuries, and even millennia – we have reasonable grounds for trusting it. In the case of breathing exercises, people over many generations have found that they seem to work; and as a result numerous more recent systems of maintaining and promoting good health include breathing exercises as part of the daily routine. Svatmarama's list of eight exercises includes all the exercises that are commonly included in other systems.

CHAPTER 7

EMOTIONS AND BREATH

It is not possible to calm the emotions if the breath is wild. You learn to control you emotions by controlling your breath.

The sun brings light to the day, and the moon brings light to the night. The breath brings light to the heart.

When you can hold your breath without effort, you can control your emotions without effort.

Emotion and breath are related to one another like milk and water. If water dries up, then a cow can no longer produce milk. If the breath is wrong, then the heart is dead.

Emotion and breath depend on one another, and function in unison. If you do not learn the control your emotions, then the senses will control your emotions. But when you control your breath, all emotional problems are overcome.

All of us know that our rate and depth and breathing are closely bound up with our emotional state. In our normal experience the causal link is from emotions to breathing: when are emotions are stirred, our breathing changes. But Svatmarama is asking us to reverse the causal link: to use breath control as a means of controlling our emotions. We can try it, and see if it works.

CHAPTER 8

INNER LIGHT AND SOUND

In order to perceive the inner light, you must learn three exercises.

The first exercise is this. Fix your eyes on some object so that your gaze becomes completely rigid and immoveable.

The second exercise is this. Raise your eyebrows slightly, half-close your eyes, and gaze at the tip of your nose.

The third exercise is this. Concentrate on the region between your eyebrows and just above them, ignoring all sounds, sights, smells and feelings.

When you have learnt to perceive the inner light, you will also perceive the inner sound. It may be like the beating of a drum, or like the gushing of a fountain.

Svatmarama's three meditation exercises are very similar to those recommended by Patanjali, and explained by Patanjali in greater depth. Other teachers of meditation have also described the inner light and sound – especially the light. There is, however, a danger that we make seeing the light and hearing the sound the test of our success in meditation; and hence, if we do not see and hear them, we feel that we have failed. Patanjali's silence on these matters assures us that meditation can reach the deepest level with no such experiences.

Tantra

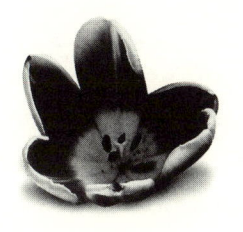

THE FABRIC OF HEALTH

INTRODUCTION

The Tantras are esoteric texts composed mainly in the first millennium CE, which circulated amongst religious sages in northern India and Tibet. *Tantra* means the 'warp of a loom'; so a Tantra contains wisdom that holds together and extends the fabric of life.

There are four Tantras concerned with health and healing. Their authorship is uncertain, and they may have been altered considerably over the centuries. But it seems likely that a Buddhist teacher in India called Padmasambhava, who lived in c8, may have written them in their original form. He was undoubtedly well-versed in Ayurvedic medicine, adopting and adapting many of its ideas. Some time later, as Buddhism spread northwards to Tibet, Padmasambhava's writings became the basis of Tibetan medicine – and to this day a Tibetan physician must learn them by heart.

The first Tantra is a short introduction. The third Tantra is a long and detailed list of diseases, their causes and symptoms. The fourth Tantra gives prescriptions for each disease. The second Tantra, from which the following extracts are taken, is mainly concerned with how to lead a healthy life.

CHAPTER 1

WIND, BILE AND PHLEGM

There are three humors: wind, bile and phlegm. Wind is weightless, cold, dry and coarse. Bile is light, hot, oily and sharp. Phlegm is heavy, tepid, moist and smooth.

There are five kinds of wind, each located in a different part of the body, and each performing different functions. Life-sustaining wind is located in the crown of the head, and runs through the brain and throat; it inhales and exhales, spits, swallows food and drink, sneezes, belches, and keeps the mind clear. Ascending wind is located in the chest, and runs through the throat, nose and mouth; it projects speech and gives physical strength. Pervading wind is located in the heart, and moves though the whole body; it enables the limbs to stretch and contract, and opens and closes the orifices. Equalizing wind is located in the stomach; it digests food. Descending wind is located in the intestines, anus, bladder and penis; it excretes waste.

There are five kinds of bile, each located in a different part of the body, and each performing different functions. Digestive bile is located in the stomach; it separates the nutritious parts of food from the waste, and it keeps the body warm. Colorful bile is located in the liver; it provides pigment to the skin and the hair. Emotional bile is located in the heart; it provides every kind of emotional response and passion. Sense bile is located in the head; it enables the senses to perceive and understand external objects. Complexion bile is located in the skin; keeps the skin clear of blemishes and gives it tone.

There are five kinds of phlegm, each located in a different part of the body, and each performing different functions. Supporting phlegm is located in the chest; it maintains the moisture level of the body. Decomposing phlegm is located in the throat; it begins the process of digesting the food, and separating nutrition from waste. Experiencing phlegm is located in the tongue and nose; it enables tastes and smells to be distinguished. Satisfying phlegm is located in the head; it enables pleasures to be enjoyed, pains to be suffered, and sleep to occur. Connecting phlegm is located in the joints, and lubricates their movement.

Good health consists in having the correct amount of every kind of humor. All diseases are caused by an excess of a particular kind of humor, or by a deficiency.

Analysis of human anatomy in recent centuries has steadily discredited many earlier descriptions of the body's inner workings, such as that propounded by Padmasambhava. But Padmasambhava, like many similar writers in both East and West, were primarily concerned with achieving balance within the body as a whole; their fundamental attitude to medicine was holistic. By contrast the medical approach that has developed in recent centuries has tended to focus on the individual parts of the body as discrete entities. Only now are we beginning seriously to question this approach, and to return to holism. So although we must reject the details of Padmasambhava's theories about wind, bile and phlegm, we can embrace the vision that lies behind the theories.

CHAPTER 2

BALANCED BEHAVIOR

Do not torment your senses, as this causes bile to accumulate; do not taste or smell things that are nasty; and do not look at or listen to things that are ugly. Do not indulge your senses, as this will cause bile to drain away.

Do not deprive yourself of sleep, and do not sleep too much; lack of sleep reduces phlegm, and excessive sleep causes phlegm to accumulate. If you miss a night's sleep, do not eat in the morning; instead sleep through the morning for half the time that you would normally sleep at night. If you sleep too little during the short nights of summer, then have a nap during the day.

Do not engage in excessive sexual activity, as this cause wind to accumulate; occasionally you may have intercourse once every two days, but once every two weeks should be normal. While the sexual urge remains, do not abstain from sexual activity, as this reduces wind.

Do not bathe too frequently as this weakens to skin; once a day is sufficient. Do not forget to bathe, as dirty and sweaty skin becomes coarse and hard.

Do not engage in excessive physical exercise, as this eventually causes the limbs and joints to grow stiff. Engage in moderate exercise each day, as this keeps the limbs agile and the brain clear.

Buddhism, the religion to which Padmasambhava adhered, preached the spiritual middle way. Padmasambhava, in his prescription for a healthy lifestyle, is advocating a physical middle way. We can look at a typical week or month of our own lives, and discern the extent to which we veer from one extreme to another. Are we sedentary for most of the time, and have occasional vigorous workouts in the gym or on the squash court? Do we deprive ourselves of food when we are busy, only to stuff ourselves when we have some leisure? Do we sleep too little through the week, and catch up at the weekend?

CHAPTER 3

SEASONAL BEHAVIOR

In the early winter the pores of the skin constrict, and wind increases. At this time you should eat foods that are sour and salty. As the nights lengthen, you will become hungry before dawn; to avoid this you should eat more oily foods.

In the late winter phlegm accumulates in the body, especially in the stomach. At this time you should eat foods that are bitter, hot and astringent. As the days lengthen, your limbs will become weary before dusk; you should undertake vigorous exercise to restore your strength.

In the early summer the heat of the sun causes phlegm to dry up. At this time you should foods that are light and cool, and you should bathe regularly in cool water.

In the rainy season bile accumulates in the body. At this time you should eat foods that are sweet, and you should fill your house with sweet fragrances.

CHAPTER 4

RESPONSIVE BEHAVIOR

If you feel inclined to vomit, do not suppress it. Suppression of vomiting causes anorexia, asthma, itching, abscesses, and eye diseases. Allow yourself to vomit; then rinse out your mouth, and fast until all feeling of sickness has passed. Inhale smoke from sandalwood.

If you feel inclined to sneeze, do not suppress it. Suppression of sneezing causes deafness, headaches, stiffness of the neck, and fractures of the jaw. Allow yourself to sneeze; then bask in bright sunlight.

If you feel inclined to yawn, do not suppress it. Suppression of yawning causes wind to accumulate.

If after exertion you are panting, do not try to stop. Suppression of panting strains the heart, and causes the brain to become confused. Inhale and exhale as much as you need.

Retire at the same time each evening, as this will enable you to sleep soundly; do not force yourself to stay awake late into the night. If you are so tense that you cannot sleep at night, massage yourself with oil. When your throat becomes clogged with phlegm, clear it. Allowing phlegm to remain in the throat causes hiccups and asthma, and weakens the heart.

Never suppress bowel movements or the urge to pass urine, as this causes toxic wastes to build up within the body, causing severe fever.

It also causes infections within the passages through which stools and urine pass.

During sexual intercourse you should emit semen when the urge is strongest; do not try to delay. And if you feel an urge to emit semen at other times, do not suppress it. Suppression of semen causes infections in the genital organs and blockages in the urinary passages.

Listen to our own bodies, and allow our bodies to do what they need to do – that is a summary of Padmasambhava's advice. It sounds simple, and children follow it naturally. But all kinds of social pressures can make us deaf to our bodies, with, according to Padmasambhava, potentially dire consequences. His list of eight forms of listening is not exhaustive; nor does he claim it to be. He is suggesting that, if we listen to our bodies in these eight particular ways, then we shall have regained the habit of listening – and we shall hear other messages as well.

CHAPTER 5

FOOD

Foods may be divided into four categories: grains, meat, oil, and vegetables.

Grains may be divided into two types: cereals and pulses. Amongst the grains rice is especially effective in reducing wind and increasing phlegm; wheat also reduces wind and reduces bile. Pulses, on the other hand, increase wind and reduce phlegm. Thus in a normal diet you should eat both grains and pulses; if you eat one without the other, you will become weak and more susceptible to illness.

Meat may be divided into two types: meat from animals that live on land, and meat from fish. Meat from animals reduces both wind and phlegm, and increases bile. Fish reduces phlegm. Thus if you eat an excessive amount of meat, your body will dry up and lose all energy. So it is safest to abstain from meat altogether; but if this is impossible, you should eat meat sparingly.

Oils of all kinds increase all three humors. Thus a small amount of oil is vital for maintaining health. But if you overload your body with oil, you quickly become obese, and hence condemn yourself to an early death. Vegetables are the perfect food. When you are deficient in any humor, they increase it; and when you have a surfeit of any humor, they reduce it. Thus they keep the three humors in perfect balance. It is best, however, to have a mixture of different vegetables; in particular, you should eat both the green vegetables that grow above the earth, and the root vegetables that grow below.

Many of us are inclined to regard vegetables almost as an optional extra; we may add to the main foods if we wish. Padmasambhava is telling us that vegetables should form the main dish – and that meat is an optional extra. As recently as the 1960s nutritionists were still emphasizing the centrality of meat to a healthy diet. Now at last they have caught up with Padmasambhava.

CHAPTER 6

DRINK

Drinks may be divided into three types: milk, water, and alcohol.

Fresh milk reduces wind and bile, and increases phlegm. But if milk is turned into curds, it loses these effects; instead it reduces phlegm. Thus you should not consume excessive amounts of either fresh milk or curds; and you should consume some of each.

Water has no effect on the humors, but purifies the body. The purest form of water is from rain; it also tastes the sweetest.

A small amount of alcohol has no effect on the humors; but a large amount imbalances them. So if you insist on consuming alcohol, you should do so in strict moderation.

In drink, as in all things, Padmasambhava advocates the middle way. But the middle way does not mean that we should have something of everything. If tobacco had been available in his time, he would probably have taught that the middle way involved excluding it altogether. The middle way can also involve the exclusion of alcohol – although, like meat, a little is allowed. We should do an honest calculation of how much alcohol we actually do drink each week. Do we really only drink it in strict moderation?

T'AI CHI

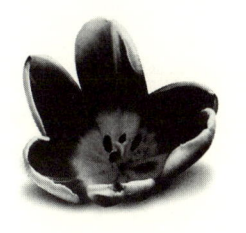

HEALTH THROUGH MOVEMENT

INTRODUCTION

T'ai chi **means 'the great energy'. It is a system of postures and movements designed to improve and maintain health.**

Its origins are hazy and, insofar as they can be discerned, rather complex. In about c3 CE a Chinese physician, Hua-Tuo, emphasized the importance of physical exercise. He argued that human beings are in reality no more than intelligent animals, but that through civilization they have lost the pliability and grace of animals; this loss is the cause of most of the illnesses and disabilities to which humans are prone. Thus he devised a regime of exercises, called 'animal games', in which humans rediscover their animal grace.

Sometime around c12 a treatise was composed, apparently based on Hua-Tuo's ideas. It is ascribed to Chang San-feng, who is often regarded as the founder of T'ai Chi; but nothing is reliably known about him. At some point T'ai Chi became a martial art; and a treatise from around c17, ascribed to Wong Chung-yua, outlines it in these terms. Wong Chung-yua is said to have wandered through China, challenging the strongest men in each place to fight him; and by confronting their physical force with softness and pliability, he trounced them all.

According to T'ai Chi all living beings have two kinds of energy. They have physical energy that gives them muscular strength; and they have a deeper and subtler energy – *chi* – that is the ultimate source of life. The primary purpose of the T'ai Chi postures and movements is to release this subtle energy. When practiced as a martial art, T'ai Chi transforms this subtle energy into *jing* – subtle power.

In the following extracts Chapters 1-3 are ascribed to Chang San-feng; Chapters 4-6 are ascribed to Wong-Chung-yua; and Chapters 7-9 are by Wu Yu-hsiang. Together they form the classic texts of T'ai Chi.

CHAPTER 1

THE PRINCIPLE OF MOVEMENT

When you move, your whole body should be light, as if it were floating. You should be aware of the connections between the various parts of the body.

The subtle energy should flow upwards through your body, and it should vibrate gently like the beat of a drum. The spirit should flow inwards to the center of your body, and it should condense there.

You should strive for perfection in every movement, allowing no faults. Every movement should be completely smooth, with no roughness; and there should be continuity between one movement and another, with no interruptions.

The subtle energy starts at the soles of the feet. It rises up through the legs, and reaches the waist, where it is controlled. From there it moves through the back to the arms, hands and fingers.

When you are drawing the subtle energy from your feet to your waist, the various parts of your body should function as one. Thus you will be able to move forwards and backwards freely, exercising complete control of your balance and your posture. If your body fails to function in unity, you will lose control of your balance and posture; and you can only gain control by examining your body with the utmost care.

You should make your mind the ultimate master of your body, guiding and directing every movement. The mind does not merely give instructions to the muscles, but infuses the muscles with intelligence.

T'ai Chi seems to require an act of faith: that such a thing as 'subtle energy' actually exists. But you can treat subtle energy as a metaphor, and T'ai Chi still remains valid: it is a metaphor for using our muscles lightly. As a matter of common experience, this feels quite different from exerting muscles to their full strength. When we push our muscles towards their limits, we find ourselves with less and less command over our bodily movements. But when we are gentle with our muscles, we can be much more precise and exact in our bodily movements – much more subtle.

CHAPTER 2

THE PRINCIPLE OF OPPOSITES

Abide always by the principle of opposites. When you move upwards, your mind should also think of downward motion. When you move forwards, your mind should also think of backward motion. When you move to the right, your mind should also think of leftward motion. So when your mind and body and moving in one direction, you mind is also moving in the opposite direction.

If you pull up a plant in order to see how well its roots are growing, you interfere with the principle of growth, and thereby threaten the plant itself. If you move in one direction without also thinking about the opposite motion, you interfere with the principle of opposites, and thereby threaten motion itself.

Distinguish clearly positive and negative energy. Positive energy is that which makes you move in a particular direction; negative energy is that which pulls you in the opposite direction. When you are aware of both positive and negative, your movements are perfect.

You may regard positive energy as the active aspect of energy, and negative energy as the passive aspect of energy. If the active and passive aspects of energy are balanced, then the various parts of the body are fully connected with one another.

Your body should move like the flow of water in a river, or the rolling of waves in the ocean.

When we exert our physical strength, we simply push our muscles in a particular direction. But when we use our muscles lightly, we have to restrain and control them. So when we move an arm lightly in a particular direction, we also prevent it from moving too quickly or heavily. For most of us in our normal daily lives we rarely need to move in this way — although certain types of artists and craftsmen do. T'ai Chi proposes that we dedicate a time each day for light movement.

CHAPTER 3

THE EIGHT POSTURES

There are eight basic postures. In practicing T'ai Chi you move from one posture to another.

The first posture is called 'ward off'. The right arm is raised, with the forearm protecting the chest. The left arm is lowered with the wrist pulled up, so the palm is facing outwards. The right leg is in front, and slightly bent at the knee. The left leg is behind, and straight at the knee.

The second posture is called 'roll-back'. The right arm is lowered, and bent at the elbow. The left arm is raised, with the forearm protecting the chest. The right leg is behind, and slightly bent at the knee. The left leg is in front, and also slightly bent at the knee.

The third posture is called 'press'. The right arm is raised with the wrist pulled up, so the palm is facing outwards. The left arm is also raised, with the hand clasping the right hand; thus the right hand is pressing on the left. The right leg is in front, and slightly bent at the knee. The left leg is behind, and straight at the knee.

The fourth posture is called 'push'. The right and left arms are raised, and slightly bent at the elbows, with the wrists pulled up, so the palms are facing outwards. The right leg is behind, and straight at the knee. The left leg is in front, and slightly bent at the knee.

The fifth posture is called 'pull'. The right and left forearms are stretched out perpendicular to the waist, with the palms facing upwards. The body is leaning backwards slightly. The right left is behind, and slightly bent at the knee. The left leg is in front, and also slightly bent at the knee.

The sixth posture is called 'split'. The right arm is lowered, and slightly bent at the elbow. The left arm is raised, and the head and body are twisted to the left. The right and left legs are parallel and wide apart, and slightly bent at the knees, with the feet pointing diagonally outwards.

The seventh posture is called 'elbow'. The right arm is lowered, and slightly bent at the elbow, with the palm facing down. The left upper arm hangs down from the shoulder, and the forearm is fully bent at the elbow, with the wrist pulled up, so the palm is facing outwards. The head and body are twisted to the right. The right leg is at the front, and bent slightly at the knee. The left leg is behind, and straight at the knee.

The eighth posture is called 'shoulder'. This position is the same as 'elbow', except that the palm of the right hand is facing inwards towards the body.

There are many other postures and movements; and these must be learnt from a proficient teacher.

Unlike the postures of Hatha Yoga, the postures of T'ai Chi require no particular suppleness or agility; any of us can manage them. And unlike the strenuous exercises performed in a gym, which build up muscles, T'ai Chi has no visible effect on the body. Indeed, the T'ai Chi exercises are utterly undemanding – and for that reason may seem a waste of time. But, according to their proponents, it is in their undemanding nature that their value lies. T'ai Chi is not designed to make us different from what we are, either physically or spiritually; it intended to make us more fully ourselves.

Through practicing these postures we gradually become more aware of our bodies, and more in control them; and at the same time we gradually become more in command of our emotions, and can thus use them more appropriately. T'ai Chi in effect claims to make us master artists and craftsmen — where we ourselves are the object of our artistry and craft.

CHAPTER 4

THE USE OF ENERGY

T'ai Chi arises from infinity and eternity. It is the source of the positive and the negative. When T'ai Chi is active, the positive and the negative separate; when T'ai Chi is passive, the positive and the negative integrate.

When you are practicing T'ai Chi, you should neither do too much or too little. You should neither rush nor hesitate. You should neither strain yourself nor allow yourself to become limp.

When you are practicing T'ai Chi, you should hold your head as if it were suspended by string from above you. In this way your back and neck will be perfectly straight, and yet also completely relaxed.

You should seek the energy for movement from the lower part of your abdomen.

The weight of your body should be immediately above your feet, so you are never straining or struggling to maintain your balance.

If the muscles on one side of the body are active, the muscles on the other side should be passive. Allow activity and passivity to flow easily from one place to another in your body.

The essence of T'ai Chi is to be able to move, and at the same time remain relaxed. That seems like a contradiction: when we relax, we are generally still and motionless. But T'ai Chi's simple prescriptions show how the contradiction can be resolved. Similar prescriptions are often given to actors and singers: if they are to sustain their performances without straining their voices and bodies, they too must move and relax at the same time.

CHAPTER 5

MARTIAL ART

When you are practicing T'ai Chi with an opponent, you should observe carefully how the opponent is moving. If the opponent is strong, do not resist that strength with strength, but yield to it. If the opponent moves in a particular direction, then you should move in that direction also. If the opponent moves faster, then you should move faster also. If the opponent moves more slowly, then you should move more slowly also.

Do not judge the opponent's movements, but match them. Once the opponent's movements have become your own, you will understand the principle of subtle energy.

When you have understood the principle of subtle energy, you can begin to acquire subtle awareness. Subtle awareness is not a theory that you can grasp with your mind; it comes through engaging in T'ai Chi over a long period. Subtle awareness does not emerge gradually; it emerges at a particular moment when you are ready.

When the opponent look upwards, you should seem tall; when the opponent looks downwards, you should seem short.
When the opponent comes towards you, then you should seem beyond reach. When the opponent retreats from you, then you should seem to be preventing any escape.

You should be so aware of your skin that you can feel even the tiniest feather brushing against your skin. You should be as sensitive to the touch of an insect as to the impact of a heavy weight. Then the opponent will not be able to control you, but you will have complete control over yourself. Indeed, if you achieve this degree of sensitivity, no force can overwhelm you.

There are countless methods and techniques in the martial arts, most of which depend on superior physical strength and speed – so the strong defeat the weak, and the fast defeat the slow. But T'ai Chi does not depend on physical ability of any kind.

With T'ai Chi only a small amount of energy is required to control the most powerful force. T'ai Chi does not confront force with force.

An old man trained in T'ai Chi can defend himself numerous opponents at once. Victory does not depend on strength and speed.

Most young boys enjoy wrestling. Usually the biggest boy with the strongest muscles wins. But sometimes a small boy with comparatively little strength can overcome even the toughest opponents. Such boys have discovered for themselves some of the secrets of T'ai Chi. Subtlety of movement, in which there is complete control, can prove far more effective than uncontrolled lunges.

CHAPTER 6

MINIMAL ENERGY

When are stationary, you should stand with your weight perfectly balanced, so that you expend minimal energy. When you move, your entire body should shift smoothly from one position to another, so that you expend minimal energy.

When you are confronting an opponent, move only as much as is necessary, and no more. Follow the flow of your opponent's movements, rather than requiring your opponent to follow the flow of your movements; in this way you will expend less energy than your opponent – and hence emerge victorious.

In order to understand how energy can be minimized, you must understand that the positive and the negative complement each other. When the positive and negative are equal, energy is conserved.

Do not try to overcome external forces with greater force. Instead, yield and submit to them; then you will be able to overcome them.

CHAPTER 7

SUBTLE ENERGY

Use your mind to direct your subtle energy. Let the subtle energy infuse your entire body, penetrating its deepest parts, even the marrow of your bones.

When you move, use your subtle energy to stimulate the motion. This means that you must circulate your subtle energy around your body, distributing it evenly. Eventually you will acquire complete control of your subtle energy, so that you determine how it functions.

Imagine that your head is suspended from the crown, so that without effort on your part your neck is stretched. This will increase the capacity of the mind to direct your subtle energy.

As you learn to use your mind to direct your subtle energy, so you will find that your subtle energy influences your mind. When subtle energy and the mind are balanced, then your body will also be balanced.

Circulating your subtle energy around your body is like guiding a thread through a pearl with many openings. If you try to hurry, or if your use any pressure you will fail. You must concentrate your mind, and yet be utterly relaxed.

While it is important to breathe correctly, do not imagine that correct breathing in itself circulates subtle energy. It is the mind alone that can circulate subtle energy – and correct breathing is an aid to the mind.

You can learn to circulate subtle energy at any time.

CHAPTER 8

SUBTLE POWER

When you practice T'ai Chi with an opponent, you must condense your subtle energy into subtle power. Subtle power enables you to overcome your opponent without physical force.

Condensing subtle energy into subtle power is like refining metal. Subtle power is pure subtle energy, and hence can never be destroyed and can never be expended.

Condensing subtle energy into subtle power is like pulling the string of a bow. Exercising subtle power is like the shooting of an arrow.

Condensing subtle energy into subtle power occurs in the spine. Thus once your mind has learnt to direct your subtle energy, you will be able to draw your subtle energy to the spine – and the condensation will then occur.

In order to draw subtle energy to the spine, you must relax your belly completely, and at the same time concentrate your mind intensely.

You cannot anticipate the moment when you will need subtle power; nor can you convert subtle energy into subtle power instantly. Thus you must regularly convert subtle energy into subtle power, and then store the subtle power.

CHAPTER 9

STILLNESS AND MOTION

When you practice T'ai Chi, you should be like an eagle. For long periods the eagle glides effortlessly on the wind. Yet it is always ready to swoop down and pluck a rabbit from the ground.

When you practice T'ai Chi, you should be like a cat. For long periods the cat lies still, watching and waiting. Yet it is always ready to leap forward and catch a mouse.

When you are still, you should be like a mountain. When you are in motion, you should be like the water of a river.

When you practice T'ai Chi, your movements should be like those of an accordion. The accordion folds and unfolds, but in itself it remains unchanged; it is both still and in motion at the same time.

When you practice T'ai Chi, you should always be soft and pliable; in this way you will be firm and strong.

If your opponent is still, you should remain still. If your opponent moves, you should move by the same amount.
You subtle power should be in a state of balance between relaxation and tension. It should be tranquil, yet also ready at all times to spring into action.

When you move, your entire body should move. When you are still, you entire body should be still.

Sometimes we are inclined to assert our superiority to animals and birds; and sometimes we ascribe to animals and birds mental and physical qualities that we have somehow lost. T'ai Chi regards cats and eagles as exemplars of the use of subtle energy and power. The effortless motion of the eagle in flight, and its occasional swoops to the ground; the light, silent steps of the cat stalking its prey, culminating in a sudden leap forward – the eagle and the cat both demonstrate the precision and control of movement that arises from being simultaneously tense and relaxed. And that is what T'ai Chi invites us to acquire for ourselves.

Muhammad

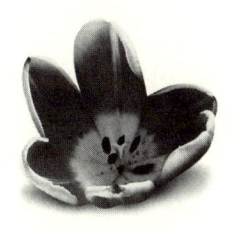

SIMPLICITY AND BALANCE

INTRODUCTION

Muhammad, the founder of Islam, made a clear distinction between the prophecies that he had received from Allah, which formed the *Quran*, and his personal ideas and opinions, which in his view had no special authority. Nonetheless his followers noted down his remarks on any and every subject; and after his death collections of his sayings, known as *hadith*, were widely circulated.

In c14, seven centuries after Muhammad's death, a Syrian scholar called Al-Jawziyya, brought together in a single volume several collections of sayings of health and healing. And a century later an Egyptian scholar called As-Suyuti brought together several more collections. It is difficult to imagine that all the sayings come from Muhammad's mouth; probably ideas from other sources were gradually added. Nonetheless the core of both books is original *hadith*.

In the following extracts the first six chapters, concerned with daily living, are from Al-Jawziyya's work. The final chapter, a compendium of different foods used as medicines, is from As-Suyuti's work; for ease of reference the foods have been put in alphabetical order according to their English names.

CHAPTER 1

PRINCIPLES OF DIET

Eating the right food is the best means of attaining and maintaining a healthy body. And if the right food can cure an illness, you should avoid every kind of artificial medicine. Indeed, when an artificial medicine cannot cure an illness, and cannot be flushed out in the normal way, it becomes a poison, and is liable to make the illness worse.

The normal cause of illness is the excess of some substance within the body that upsets the body's natural balance. This excess can arise for five reasons. First, you may eat too much. Secondly, you may eat too frequently, consuming each meal before the previous meal has been digested. Thirdly, you may eat food that is deficient in particular nutrients, so the food is unbalanced. Fourthly, you may eat food that is slow and difficult to digest, so that it remains undigested in the stomach for a long time. Fifthly, you may eat opposing types of food in the same meal.

Good food has three essential qualities. First, it is wholesome, containing nutrients that are beneficial to the body. Secondly, it is light, so that it does not strain the body; thus it should not contain excessive fat. Thirdly, it is easy to digest.

There are three levels of diet: a necessary diet; a sufficient diet; and an excessive diet. A necessary diet is that which maintains life, but does not provide strength and energy. An excessive diet gradually destroys life by forcing the body to carry excess weight. Thus you should have a sufficient diet, that is more than what is necessary, but less than what is excessive.

Muhammad regards wrong eating as the main source of illness. It is a bold claim, and seems to contradict our modern understanding: we ascribe most illnesses to bacterial or viral infections. And modern medical treatment is mostly based on this understanding. Yet it fails to explain why one person falls prey to a particular illness, while another remains immune, even though both have the same degree of exposure. Diet is manifestly an important factor in determining our relative immunity. And Muhammad's list of five types of wrong eating seems comprehensive.

CHAPTER 2

BALANCED DIET

You should eat a variety of food, and not eat a particular kind of food over a long period. Indeed, if your diet is monotonous, it will harm your digestion, and weaken its ability to absorb other types of food in the future.

You should eat the foods that occur naturally in the area where you are living. You should not eat foods imported from far away. By eating local foods your diet will be in harmony with the climate, the atmosphere and all the other aspects of the environment.

You should balance heat and moisture in your diet. When you are consuming something hot and dry, ensure that you are also eating something that is cool and moist. If you have insufficient moisture in your diet, the organs of your body will cease to function.

You should balance the tastes of your food. When you are eating something bland, you should eat with it something that has a strong flavor. Do not, for example, eat bread alone; you may perhaps dip it in vinegar. Do not eat a spicy dish without also eating something easy on the palate.

You should ensure that in each meal the various foods and dishes are digested at a similar rate. You should not mix dishes that are easy to digest with dishes that are hard to digest. For example, you should not eat broiled and roasted food in the same meal; nor should you eat milk with eggs or meat.

You should food in its season; do not try to preserve food over a long period. The best food of all is fruit in its season. Fresh fruit contains many nutrients, and cures numerous illnesses. It also contains both the moisture and the heat of the land in which it grew and the season in which it ripened; so it has the perfect balance of heat and moisture.

Food should be cooked slowly at a sufficient distance from the fire. If food is held close to the fire, the exterior of the food will be fully cooked while the interior is still raw. And do not reheat food, as this is liable to poison you.

If you dislike a particular food, then you should avoid eating it; your dislike is a sign that the food would be bad for your body. And if, when you start to consume a particular dish, you start to feel queasy, then you should set the dish aside.

Most of us find ourselves in agreement with most of Muhammad's dietary advice. But two pieces of advice in particular are likely to trouble us: to eat local food; and to eat food in season. Our shops are filled with foods from all over the world, and the choice remains virtually unchanged through the year. The basis of Muhammad's advice is that our bodies adapt to the local environment and climate; and so local, seasonal foods are likely to suit our bodily needs. To some degree this view is undermined by another feature of modern life, our mobility; many of us move several times in the course of our lives. Nonetheless our bodies respond remarkably quickly to local conditions; and while Muhammad's advice may not be applied dogmatically, we may still have a preference for foods produced near home.

CHAPTER 3

METHOD OF EATING

The best posture at meals is to sit on the floor. You may be cross-legged, or sit on one leg while leaning on the other, or stretch out both legs in front of you. Your whole body should be relaxed as you eat

You should not eat standing up, as this will tend to make your body tense, and hence hinder your digestion. You should eat lying on your stomach, as this prevents the stomach from absorbing the food. You should not recline to one side, as this restricts the flow of food through your body.

Although you may bend over when you put food in your mouth, you should sit upright when chewing and swallowing food. This enables the food to pass easily down your gullet.

Some wealthy people like to recline on pillows while they are eating, resting their arms on bolsters. This causes no physical problems, but is a sign of arrogance. Since food is a divine gift, it should be eaten in a posture of humility.

It is best to eat with three fingers. If you use five fingers, you are liable to put too much in your mouth at once. If you use a fork and spoon, the process of eating is so easy that you are liable to eat too much.
In order to benefit fully from the nutrients in your food, you should take pleasure in eating. Thus eat slowly enough to enjoy the full flavor of every morsel.

Do not miss a meal, even if you are on a long journey or engaged in some demanding occupation. At every mealtime consumer something, even if it only a handful of dates. If the stomach is ready to digest food, but has nothing to digest, it will poison itself.

Muhammad treats the eating of a meal almost as a religious ritual. But unlike a religious ritual, where the movements and gestures are mainly symbolic, the proper way of consuming food is, according to Muhammad, severely practical: if we conduct ourselves wrongly at meals, we shall suffer dire consequences. His rules can be encapsulated in two simple principles: eating should be slow and relaxed. In the modern context he is asking us the reject the entire culture of fast food.

CHAPTER 4

DRINK

Do not drink while you are eating as this enfeebles to digestive process. Wait for some time after a meal before drinking.

Every morning drink cold honey sweetened with a spoonful of honey. Honey both cleanses the body, and purifies the body of any toxins. It dissolves any obstructions in the bladder, liver and kidney. It warms up the stomach, and so prepares it to digest food. It helps the bowels to move. And it stimulates the appetite.

While water sweetened with honey is beneficial, water sweetened with sugar is harmful. Excessive sugar causes the body to age prematurely, while honey keeps the body youthful.

Do not drink water by lapping it with your tongue from a pond, while lying on your stomach; and do not drink water from your hand. Drink from a cup or a waterskin. In general you should not drink while standing up, as this will not fully slake your thirst; it is best to drink while sitting down.

Do not drink quickly, as this strains the liver and the heart. Drinking quickly can be especially dangerous in hot weather, as the shock of the cold liquid can cause your windpipe to contract, so that you choke. Drink slowly, taking a breath between each gulp.

Drink milk every day. You may drink it fresh, or fermented as yogurt; and you may dilute it with water. Milk contains many nutrients that benefit the body. When a herd has been grazing on lavender, its milk is especially good.

In the Bible God promises the Hebrew people 'a land of milk and honey.' Muhammad, who was very familiar with Biblical teaching, regards milk and honey as the two finest forms of nutrition available to us. If we link this with his belief in local foods, he is advising us to drink milk from local herds, and to eat honey from local bees. Since bees make honey from pollen, and since pollen induces several allergic reactions including hay fever, many believe that local honey is the best protection from these reactions.

CHAPTER 5

CLOTHES AND SHELTER

Dress in loose clothing. Wear a long shirt with sleeves that hang just short of the wrist. And have an outer garment that hangs down just short of the ankles. Always wear a turban outdoors to keep your head cool in hot weather and warm in cold weather.

Do not aspire to live in some grand mansion. A home has only three purposes: to protect you from the weather; to provide privacy; and to provide a place to relax and sleep. A small, simple house with a few articles of furniture can fulfill these – and you should want nothing more.

To ensure that your house is free of disease, it should be built on clean, dry land; it should be well ventilated; and some pleasant perfume should be sprayed within it.

CHAPTER 6

SLEEP AND EXERCISE

Retire early, so that you sleep during the first half of the night. Rise soon after the middle of the night, and spend a long period in silent thought and meditation. Then retire again, and have a short sleep before dawn. As the sun rises, you will awake refreshed in body and in soul.

You may have a short nap during the day if you feel tired. But do not sleep under the sun, as this may cause cancerous growths and other hidden diseases.

In maintaining good health, and in curing illnesses, physical exercise is as important as food. Have a regular routine in which you exercise the limbs, the lungs and heart, and the voice.

While wrong eating is the main cause of illness, the wrong environment and daily regime can also, according to Muhammad, be highly dangerous. Muhammad himself, although he eventually became ruler of almost all Arabia, always lived very simply, wearing the normal loose garments of the Arab nomad, sleeping in a mud hut, and often engaging in manual work. And although he died in his early 60s, he was remarkably fit and healthy until his final illness. At first sight his sleeping routine seems extremely tough. But in fact it accords with two aspects of our common experience. First, a few hours of deep sleep is very refreshing; and we can only ensure this by going to bed at roughly the same time each night. Secondly, one or two short naps through the day are more effective in maintaining alertness than prolonging sleep at night. Some enlightened companies now provide facilities for their employees to lie down in the middle of the day; as a result productivity in the afternoon rises steeply.

CHAPTER 7

FOODS AS MEDICINES

In addition to providing nutrition, many foods may also be used as medicines.

Almonds help to dissolve stones in the kidney and gall bladder.

Aniseed soothes internal pains and dispels wind. Nursing mothers should take it to help the flow of milk; and men suffering impotence should take it to help the flow of semen.

Apples strengthen the heart. They are also an antidote to malicious emotions, and tend to make people feel more kindly and compassionate. But only sweet apples should be eaten, sour apples, even if they are sweetened with sugar or honey, harm the memory.

Apricots are excellent for the stomach. They should first be dried; and then, shortly before being eaten, they should be soaked in water.

Asparagus relieves blockages in the kidney, and helps back pain. It also makes labor easier for women giving birth.

Beans of all kinds are an excellent source of nourishment, helping to prevent all kinds of illnesses. They are liable to cause flatulence; but this can be prevented if they are eaten with thyme, olive oil and salt.

Butter aids the digestion, and relieves dry coughs. It also reduces the appetite. So if someone is inclined to overeat, a small amount of butter at meals reduces this tendency. Or on a long journey when food is scarce, butter stops the pangs of hunger.

Chamomile is a mild laxative, and it dispels wind; it also a diuretic, helping the flow of urine.

Carrots increase the sexual urge, and produce a good supply of semen.

Cheese is an aphrodisiac, stimulating the sexual urge. It is also good for ulcers of the stomach and bowel, and it alleviates diarrhea. But it is liable to make you excessively fat, so it should only be eaten in small quantities.

Coffee is good for dysentery and enteritis. It helps the mind to think faster, and engenders wisdom.

Coriander seeds are a helpful in treating all diseases except cancer.

Currants help to warm a cold body, and are very nutritious. They drive away fatigue; they calm anger and relieve stress; they increase concentration; they expel phlegm; they increase the pleasure of sexual intercourse; and they clear the complexion. But their seeds can irritate the stomach, and cause pain; so they should be eaten sparingly.

Dates help to balance the temperament. In particular, they calm anger, and so reduce the tendency in some people to sudden rage.

Eggs are good for coughs and hoarseness, and they are also an aphrodisiac. They should be soft-boiled, since hard-boiled eggs produce wind.

Figs pass swiftly through the intestines, and hence act as a laxative. They also clear phlegm, and hence relieve chronic coughs. Fresh figs are better than dried figs; and they should be ripe and peeled. They are even more effective when they are eaten with almonds and walnuts.

Garlic dispels wind. It is good for rheumatism and arthritis. And it lifts the hearts of those who are depressed.

Grapes are highly nutritious; and the best grapes are the last to be harvested. Eating grapes regularly helps to protect the body against disease.

Honey is the best of all medicines. There is no illness that honey does not help to cure. It also slows down the process of ageing. And if a person has developed a taste for unhealthy foods, a regular lick of honey restores the taste for healthy foods.

Leeks help to prevent piles. But if they are eaten before going to bed, they induce nightmares.

Lettuce contains more nourishment than any other vegetable. It reduces fever. But it dried up semen, and reduces sexual desire. And eating lettuce every day weakens the eyesight.

Lime juice, when drunk with sugar, protects the body against disease, and also stimulates the appetite. It helps to stop vomiting and diarrhea.

Lupins, when eaten with honey, they kill worms.

Hazel nuts slow down the digestion and create bile, so the digestive system operates more efficiently. They also make the brain grow, and so increase intelligence.

Marjoram frees blockages in the brain, and dissolves catarrh.

Milk purifies the body, increases the production of semen, relaxes the bowels, lifts depression, stimulates the brain, improves the complexion, and alleviates itching. But the milk of any animal with a longer gestation period than that of humans should be avoided.

Mustard stimulates the brain and aids the memory. It also reduces phlegm. But too much mustard over a long period can cause blindness.

Myrtle stops diarrhea; and both its taste and fragrance soothe a headache.

Olive oil can help to cure every kind of disease and relieves every kind of pain; and regular consumption of olive oil strengthens the heart, makes the blood flow smoothly.

Onions stimulate the production of semen. They also reduce the production of phlegm, keeping the nasal passages clear. Sniffing an onion reduces nausea.

Parsley makes the breath smell sweet. Pregnant women should eat it, as it helps their offspring to be intelligent.

Peaches relax the stomach and ease the bowels. It is better to eat peaches before a meal rather than after one.

Pistachio nuts are remarkable in their effects. The outer skin stops vomiting and diarrhea, while the kernel, when eaten with egg yolk, fortifies the heart and invigorates the limbs.

Poppies relax the mind and the body; so, when someone is suffering great stress and insomnia, they induce slumber. But they should not be used frequently in this manner.

Pumpkins calm the troubled mind, and relieve coughs and fevers.

Radishes help the stomach to digest other foods, but are themselves hard to digest; so they should be eaten sparingly. They clear blockages in the liver.

Rhubarb dissolves blockages in the liver, and it relieves chronic fevers.

Rice is the most nourishing grain after wheat. It is good for the temperament, making a person calmer and less prone to anxiety, and inducing sweet dreams. It also helps to reduce swellings.

Unfortunately it is liable to cause constipation; but if it is eaten with milk, this danger is reduced.

Salt improves the complexion, while lack of salt reduces energy. But if it is eaten excessively, it causes itching.

Senna can help to cure every kind of disease except cancer. In particular, it is extremely effective in relieving constipation.

Spinach acts as a laxative, but can irritate the throat and chest.

Sugar relaxes the stomach, so helps to relieve indigestion. Brown sugar is more soothing than white.

Tamarisk seeds thicken the blood. So when the skin is cut in an accident or in battle, the bleeding stops quickly and the wound soon heals. But if they are consumed in excess, they may weaken the heart.

Thyme expels wind, and helps the stomach to digest heavy food. It also improves the complexion, and, when taken as a drink, kills worms and tapeworms.

Vinegar is good for inflammation of the stomach, and it counteracts phlegm. It should not, however, be taken early in the morning, as this reduces sexual potency.

Walnuts, when they are eaten with honey, are good for sore throats.

Water is not only essential in itself, but also enables the nutrients of food to pass into the blood. Flowing water is better than still water; and water flowing over earth is better than water flowing over stones.

Wheat is the most nourishing of all grains. It is hot, and halfway between wet and dry. It should never be eaten raw, as raw wheat harms the intestines and causes wind. Flour should be used on the same day that it has been ground.

Razi

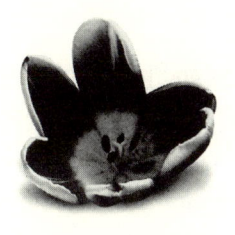

SPIRITUAL MEDICINE

INTRODUCTION

Razi, a Muslim physician and philosopher, wrote a monograph and measles that guided the treatment of those diseases across the world for eight centuries. He was also one of the first writers to stress the importance of mental health, and wrote a pioneering work on 'spiritual medicine'. He explored some common mental problems, such as anxiety, obsession, and excessive anger, and emphasized the importance of counseling.

Born in Iran near modern Tehran, he traveled to Baghdad where he studied medicine. After several years practicing as a physician he was invited by the caliph to found and direct a hospital. Later in his life he moved to Herat in modern Afghanistan, where he died in 925 CE.

CHAPTER 1

REASON OVER PASSION

You should consult reason in every situation and on all matters. You should accord it the highest respect, and trust its conclusions.

In particular, you must not give any passion mastery over reason. Passion blemishes reason; it clouds reason, diverting it from its proper path and purpose.

No, you must learn to control and govern your passion. If you succeed in this, your reason will become pure and clear; it will illuminate you with its light.

Razi is not urging us to suppress our passions, and then pretend to ourselves that they do not exist. He does not want us to drain ourselves of all emotions, so we become entirely cerebral, like computers that happen to be made of flesh. He is asking us to reflect rationally on our emotional responses, asking which are positive and beneficial, and which are negative and harmful.

CHAPTER 2

THE ROLE OF A COUNSELOR

You are naturally inclined to love yourself: you approve and admire your own actions, and you look with favor on you own character and conduct. Thus you are unlikely to have an honest view of your own unhealthy attitudes and habits – and this makes it difficult for you to change those attitudes and habits.

Therefore you need a person of insight – a counselor – whom you see frequently, and whom you can trust. This counselor should ask you many questions about yourself, gathering information about your attitudes and habits. You must answer these questions honestly, indicating that you are grateful for the opportunity to reveal all aspects of yourself, bad as well as good. You must not be shy, nor should you give trite and easy answers; and you should hold nothing back.

Eventually your counselor will begin to tell you about yourself. When this happens, you should not show any sorrow or shame. On the contrary, you should seem to rejoice at what you hear, and indicate your eagerness for more. If you think that your counselor is concealing something about yourself for fear of offending you, or is being too moderate in expressing disapproval, you should insist that you wish to hear the whole truth about yourself. Equally, if you feel your counselor has been excessive in expressing disapproval or disgust, you must on no account fly into a rage.

The task of your counselor is slow and unending. Moreover, bad attitudes and habits, which you thought you had overcome, are apt to reassert themselves. So you must ask your counselor time and time again to report on your spiritual and emotional state. You may also encourage your counselor to ask neighbors, colleagues and friends about you – what they find in you to praise, and what they find to blame.

If you have such a counselor, hardly any of your bad attitudes and habits will remain hidden from you; even the smallest and most secret bad attitude and habit will be laid bare.

You will now have nothing to fear from enemies who take delight in exposing your weaknesses and vices. You enemies will be able to reveal nothing that you do not already know; so you cannot be humiliated. On the contrary, you will be able to assure them that you are already striving to overcome the vices that they have exposed; and you will express gratitude to them for helping you in this. Thus you will treat your enemies as additional counselors, and derive benefit from them.

Razi's conception of a good counselor is very different from that prevailing today. We expect a counselor to be empathetic, encouraging, and understanding, but rarely directly critical. For Razi, by contrast, pointing out bad habits and attitudes is the counselor's main function. Razi's conception of how should receive counsel is also at odds with modern notions. We regard it as vital to be completely open and honest with the counselor, expressing our feelings without reserve. Razi says that we should always show pleasure at what the counselor says, even when we do not feel it, in order to make it easier for the counselor to tell us our faults. Of course, none of us actually wants a critical counselor. But is that the sort of counselor we need? And, of course, none of us wants to have the responsibility of enabling our counselor to be brutally frank. But should we take that responsibility, for our own good?

CHAPTER 3

CONCEIT

Since you are in love with yourself, you are inclined to overestimate your own strengths, and underestimate your own weaknesses; equally you are inclined to underestimate the strengths of others, and overestimate their weaknesses. If you allow this attitude to grow freely, with any restraint, it becomes conceit.

The irony of conceit is that it leads to the diminution of the strengths that are the original objects of conceit. Conceited people never seek to enhance the strengths about which they are conceited; and their conceit makes them deaf to the advice and guidance of others. Thus, if they are conceited about their work, they think it can never be improved. And as they cease trying to enhance their strengths, those strengths diminish.

To overcome conceit you should not judge yourself against those who lack the strengths about which you feel conceited. Instead you should judge yourself against those who excel. In this way you will observe things day by day that will reduce your estimate of yourself, and increase your admiration of others.

Our tendency towards conceit is precisely the reason why we need a counselor – or at least a spouse or close friend – who is willing to be severe with us.

CHAPTER 4

ENVY

Envy consists in taking pleasure in the injuries that befall others, and resenting anything that occurs to their advantage. Envy is worse that miserliness: misers do not want to give anything of their own to others, whereas envious people do not want others to receive anything.

Consider those who are the objects of your envy. If you are gripped by envy, you believe that other people are intensely happy, and enjoy great wealth and luxury; and you think that their happiness and wealth are undeserved. But, if you were to inform yourself about their history and condition, you would probably find yourself quite mistaken. Certainly they may experience periods of happiness, but these are probably both transient and infrequent; and their wealth probably causes them as much anxiety as it does comfort.

You will probably then conclude that quiet contentment and modest wealth are preferable to their lot – and these are within your grasp. In short, envy is based on ignorance; and this ignorance is easily dispelled.

CHAPTER 5

ANGER

Anger has been put into all animals, including humans, as a stimulus to repel those who threaten injury, or to take revenge on those who have already caused injury; thus anger is essential both for survival and for justice. But when anger goes beyond its proper bounds, it both threatens survival and infringes justice. Try to recall incidents when your own anger has been disproportionate, and thence has caused harm.

When your anger is aroused, you should do nothing immediately; you should give yourself time to reflect and deliberate. If you conclude that your anger is proportionate, then you may act on it. But if you conclude that it is disproportionate, then you must suppress it.

Moreover, in moments of anger do let arrogance fuel your fury. Do not think yourself superior to the person who has enraged you, because that will make it even more difficult to control your anger. If your anger is proportionate, and if you remain humble, then you will act justly.

Envy and anger are the two main emotions that put a barrier between ourselves and others, and thence make love impossible. They intrude from time to time in every relationship, even a close and happy marriage; and this tends to occur when we least expect it. So Razi is advising us to be constantly vigilant. The effort of overcoming envy and anger is entirely internal and invisible, consisting of profound and honest introspection;

and it is likely to be quite painful. Indeed, Razi is making clear to us that, unless we are willing and able to become uncomfortable with ourselves, we can never become masters of ourselves; and unless we become masters of ourselves, we shall never enjoy the pleasure of truly intimate and loving relationships.

CHAPTER 6

WORRY AND ANXIETY

When you are threatened by some misfortune, or you are faced with some new challenge, it is quite rational to feel anxious. But you may experience anxiety that is quite disproportionate to the external cause. This makes you less able to cope with misfortune or rise to challenges – and so you become anxious about your own anxiety.

When anxiety grips your mind and body, strive to relax. You may engage in amusing and entertaining activities that divert your mind and exercise your body. Or you may sit down and meditate, consciously striving to release the tension within you.

In times of tranquility consider the folly of your anxiety. In truth you have great capacity to cope with misfortune, and you are able to rise to challenges with great energy and intelligence. Thus you will realize that anxiety is the opposite vice to conceit: it arises from underestimating, rather than overestimating, your strengths. And it is just as bad.

To those who are naturally phlegmatic and optimistic, anxiety and worry are just plain stupid; and they frequently tell their anxious friends that worrying about something is useless. In fact, of course, it is perfectly rational to worry about potential dangers, since it makes us more careful in avoiding them. But it is utterly irrational and harmful to worry about false dangers, trivial problems, or future events over which we have no control. Razi regards irrational worry as a vicious circle that we need to break.

CHAPTER 7

MANNERISMS

You may have several mannerisms, such as fidgeting, of which you are barely aware, but which cause irritation to others. In order to rid yourself of these mannerisms, you must come to feel ashamed of them; shame is the string by which your mind can control your hands and fingers.

Shame arises from seeing yourself as others see you. So in order to instill shame within yourself, you must encourage others consistently to point out your mannerisms, and to express their disdain and contempt for them.

Compared with many other bad habits, irritating mannerisms are trivial. Yet by learning to overcome them, you will gain wisdom and strength in overcoming habits and attitudes that are far worse.

CHAPTER 8

OBSESSION

People sometimes develop an obsession over something. The most common object of obsession is cleanliness, in which washing becomes a ritual that must be performed with absurd frequency.

If you become obsessed with cleanliness, you can overcome in three stages. First, tell yourself frequently that your obsession arises from confusion between the material and the mental realms. Cleanliness is a matter of bodily health and comfort, whereas you have turned it into a mental requirement.

Secondly, ensure that you do not justify your obsession on religious grounds. True religion is concerned with inner purity, not with external cleanliness.

Thirdly, tell yourself that the root of your obsession is squeamishness about dirt. Squeamishness is a passion; and like every other passion it must be made subject to reason.

People with very serious obsessions would say that Razi's advice is inadequate, and that they require expert medical treatment over a long period. But Razi is alluding to the level of obsession to which many of us are prone: we can continue to function quite adequately, but the quality of our lives is impaired. He understands that some obsessions express themselves in religious terms, and may even be instilled by religious activity. In such cases we need to be freed – redeemed – from religion.

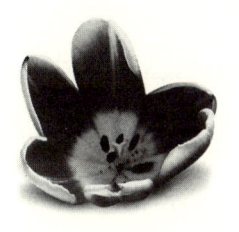

Hildegard

Body and Soul

INTRODUCTION

Hildegard, who was born in western Germany in 1098, was one of the towering geniuses of the medieval period. She was a forceful monastic leader who asserted the rights of women; she was a composer whose music has been rediscovered in the present age; she was a great mystic who described her visions in vivid prose; and towards the end of her life she was a popular preacher.

She was also deeply interested in human health, and wrote an extensive work on the subject. Much of this work is taken with enumerating the various herbal remedies that were used at the time, and which in her view were effective. However, her underlying interest was the relationship between the body and the soul – and thence between sickness of the body and the state of the soul.

CHAPTER 1

THE FOUR ELEMENTS

The four elements of fire, air, water and earth combine in different ways to form every material object and living being in the universe, including the human body. They are found in every organ of the body, and enable every organ to function.

From fire we derive the heat in our bodies, from which all energy comes, and by which we have sight. From air we derive breath, which enables our bodies to move, and by which we can hear. From water we derive the blood that is the fount of life itself. And from earth we derive the muscle and bone that form the substance of our bodies.

If the elements combine correctly across the land, then we have bountiful harvests. But sometimes they fail to combine correctly: there may be excessive rain, causing the earth to flood; or the may be excessive warmth, causing the earth to dry up; or there may be excessive wind, causing the crops and trees to blow down. When this occurs, the harvest is poor, and people suffer hunger and starvation.

Similarly, if the elements combine correctly in the body, then the body enjoys good health. But sometimes a body has excessive moisture, excessive wind, excessive blood, or excessive flesh; then that body suffers pain and illness.

The idea that there are four elements, fire, air, water and earth, derives from classical Greek thought. And although we now know it to be false, it remains a powerful idea which modern poet still use as a metaphor. In analyzing the body and its potential ills in terms of the four elements, Hildegard creates a powerful image. And although we cannot take it literally, we can treat it as a kind of narrative – a way of thinking about the body. And it leads to the conclusion that health consists of achieving balance between all the body's elements.

CHAPTER 2

THE SOUL

A human being is both a body and a soul. While the body is made of the four elements, the soul is made of divine substance.

The eyes are the windows to the soul. When the eyes are clear and shining, it is a sign that the soul is in good health; and when the soul is in good health, the mind is intelligent, quick and sharp. When the eyes are cloudy and dull, it is a sign that the soul is sick; and when the soul is sick, the mind is confused, slow and blunt.

The health of the body depends on the health of the soul; if the soul is sick, then the body becomes sick also. Thus if you wish to see whether a body is liable to fall sick, look into the eyes. If the eyes have become cloudy and dull, then the body will soon fall sick – even though they may be no symptoms at present. If the eyes appear so cloudy and dull as to be lifeless, then the body is likely to die soon. But if the eyes are bright and clear, then the body is likely to remain healthy.

There are three causes for sickness of the soul, and they should be clearly distinguished. The first cause is that the soul is filled with evil thoughts and feelings; the second cause is that the soul is burdened with the evils of others; the third cause is that the soul is preparing to pass from the present life to a future life. The first kind of sickness of the soul is a matter of the gravest concern; and it can only be cured by repentance. The second cause arises from great spiritual sensitivity, and may motivate acts of great compassion and generosity. The third cause is entirely outside human control.

Although Hildegard was a devout Christian, the notion of the soul is not found in early Christian thinking; Christianity took it over from ancient Greek philosophers such as Plato. Many people today find it problematic. But in this context Hildegard is discussing various kinds of mental disturbance, which are matters of common experience. And in her first two sicknesses of the soul she makes an important distinction between forms of mental disturbance that are negative, and those that are positive. All kinds of mental disturbance are unpleasant; we should all like to enjoy constant peace and tranquility. But mental disturbance can sometimes prompt us into acts of great generosity, compassion and courage; and artistic creativity often emerges from a disturbed mind. So Hildegard is challenging us to embrace and welcome some forms of mental turmoil, using our inner anguish to good purpose.

CHAPTER 3

DREAMS

Dreams occur within the soul. They provide a means whereby people can gain insights into both the body and the soul.

Dreams may reveal in stark terms a soul's motives and desires. If a soul has malign motives and desires, then the person will have dreams in which evil triumphs – yet, far from bringing pleasure and satisfaction, this triumph induces fear and guilt. If a soul has benign motives and desires, then the person will have dreams in which goodness triumphs, inducing contentment and joy.

Dreams may reveal imbalances in the elements that form the body, and thus may foretell a disease. If the elements are imbalanced, the person may dream of accidents and battles in which the body is injured; and the nature and location of the injury may indicate the nature and location of the impending illness. In such cases it is wise to seek a physician immediately, since sicknesses can most easily be cured before the symptoms appear.

Dreams may reveal important moral and spiritual issues. People are often so preoccupied with material concerns during the day that they ignore moral and spiritual matters. But dreams remind people that moral and spiritual welfare is more important than material welfare. And when they have received such a reminder, they should act on it – otherwise they will jeopardize the health of their souls.

Ever since psychology emerged as a distinct discipline in the late nineteenth century, psychologists have been debating how dreams should be understood and interpreted. It is a debate that is unlikely ever to reach a definitive conclusion. Nonetheless most of us have found from time to time that a dream seems to indicate something about ourselves and our circumstances that turns out to be true. Hildegard suggests three ways in which dreams may correspond with the truth; and thus she offers us a kind of checklist for interpretation. So when we awake with a dream still vivid in our minds, we can run through the checklist. Does the dream tell us anything about our desires that we have been partially hiding from ourselves? May the dream indicate the early stages of some illness? Or is the dream some kind of moral warning?

CHAPTER 4

THE FOUR TEMPERAMENTS

There are four temperaments: the sanguine temperament; the phlegmatic temperament; the choleric temperament; and the melancholic temperament. These suffuse both the body and the soul.

People with a sanguine temperament have heavy bones, and are inclined to plumpness. They are subtle in their thinking, they are pessimistic in their outlook, and their emotions are gentle and easily controlled.

People with a phlegmatic temperament have light bones, and are also inclined to plumpness. They are practical in their thinking, they are optimistic in their outlook, and their emotions are gentle and easily controlled.

People with a choleric temperament have heavy bones, and tend to remain slender. Their thoughts tend to be logical and straight, they are optimistic in their outlook, and their emotions are passionate and hard to control.

People with a melancholic temperament have light bones, and then to remain slender. Their thoughts range freely, they are pessimistic in their outlook, and their emotions are passionate and hard to control.

People should recognize their own temperament, and live in accordance with it. If they delude themselves, imagining that they have a different temperament, they cause themselves – and those around them – great misery and suffering.

Hildegard adopted her notion of four temperaments, like that of four elements, from ancient Greek thought. Most people have a mixture of temperamental tendencies. Nonetheless it is striking how many of us have a single dominant tendency; and it is even more striking how closely our physical characteristics seem to conform to our temperament. By using this ancient classification of temperament Hildegard is giving us a simple means of coming to understand ourselves more fully. She is also making an important spiritual point: we should not try to change our natural selves, as many religious teachers have urged; rather we should accept – and love – ourselves as we are.

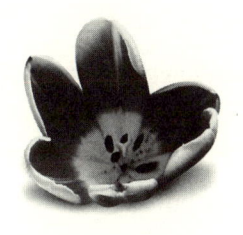

Andrew Boorde

HEATH THROUGH MIRTH

INTRODUCTION

Born in 1490 in southern England, Andrew Boorde was encouraged by his parents to become a Carthusian monk, spending almost the entire day in solitude and eating only bread and a few vegetables. Then he was appointed a bishop, while remaining under monastic discipline. But he was utterly miserable and dogged by sickness. Finally his body and spirit rebelled: he abandoned his monastic vows, and embarked on a tour of Europe, consulting physicians and sages on the means of attaining health and happiness.

When he returned to England, he became a physician himself, and soon acquired many of the leading figures of the country as patients. He very rarely prescribed medicines. Instead, he looked for the sources of illness in the way in which people led their daily lives – their diet, their pattern of sleeping, their occupations, and the location and design of the house in which they lived.

In 1542 he published his ideas in a short book entitled *The Dietary of Health* – the first medical book written in the English language. His central theme is the importance of 'mirth', by which he meant both health and happiness; and he was convinced that it was impossible to have one without the other.

CHAPTER I

MIRTHFUL HEART

The best way to remain in good health, and to avoid disease, is to have a contented and happy heart, full of mirth. Do not allow inward anger and resentment to infect your heart. Do not be unduly introspective, reflecting on your own sins and faults; when you observe yourself doing wrong, confess the sin, make amends - and forget all about it. Do not work throughout the day, but break the day with periods in which to relax and to converse with friends. Do not be unduly ambitious; attempt only those things which you have the natural ability to achieve.

The heart is the central organ in your body. It gives life to all the other organs, and is the source of your vital spirits. There is nothing that comforts and strengthens the heart so much as honest mirth, stimulated by good company. Mirth comes in many ways. Principally it comes when you show love and generosity towards neighbors. It also comes when you gather with friends to be merry, laughing and joking without swearing and slandering others. Musical instruments bring mirth; and so do good food and drink.

Has a doctor ever asked you whether you are happy and contented? When you have fallen ill, have you ever asked yourself whether sadness and discontent may be a cause? We do not readily make a link between happiness and health. Yet we know from experience that those enduring an acrimonious break-up of a partnership are prone to illness; and when one half of a long and happy marriage dies, the other half often dies quite soon afterwards. A broken heart is a dangerous condition. Even the trauma of moving house can set off a bout of minor ailments.

CHAPTER 2

A MIRTHFUL HOUSE

The most important factor affecting your health and well-being is the place where you live. You do not need a great mansion or luxurious furniture. A simple cottage, warm in the winter, cool in the summer, and dry at all times, is quite sufficient; indeed it is better, because keeping it in good repair will cause little expense and anxiety. Your cottage should have access to clear, clean water; bad water is a major cause of disease. Above all your cottage, and the garden surrounding it, should be pleasing to the eye, and hence bring contentment to the heart.

There is nothing that is so poisonous to the body as foul air - except poison itself. Air surrounds and envelops us; we take it into our bodies with every breath; we depend on air for life itself, as fish depend on water. Clean, pure air comforts the heart, clears the brain, stimulates the muscles and strengthens the nerves. Foul corrupt air sickens the heart, confuses the brain, makes the muscles grow limp, and causes the nerves to jangle. So in choosing a place to live, ensure that the area has good air. And when building your house, ensure there is plenty of ventilation, so that the air you breathe out is quickly dispersed. Also clean the chamber pots as soon as you rise in the morning, so that their smell does not linger.

There are two ways to expel foul air that has accumulated in your house. You may also use these methods to prevent foul air from accumulating, and to ensure that the atmosphere is always pure. The first is to take dried rosemary, bay leaves, and marjoram, and to mix and grind them into a powder. Put some burning pieces of wood or coal into a metal container, and sprinkle the powder onto them, causing a fragrant smoke to arise. Carry the container to every room in the house, letting the smoke fill every corner. The second method is to make pomanders of nutmeg and thyme. Soak the nutmegs in rosewater, and then take them out and allow them to dry. The nutmegs and thyme should be put in little dishes, or boxes with holes in the lid, and placed in every room.

When you build a house, consider carefully the way it faces. If it faces south, it will catch the south wind, which is warm and muggy, carrying many diseases. If it faces east, it will catch the east wind, which is fresh and fragrant. If it faces west, it will catch the west wind, which can be either warm or cold. If it faces north, it will catch the north wind, which is clean and pure. Therefore let the windows of your house face north or east - or, best of all, northeast.

In designing your house, observe which way the land slopes. Put the parlor and the bedrooms at the highest level, the kitchen and pantry at a lower level, and the privies at the lowest. The reason for this is that the waste from the kitchen will drain away from the main living quarters, and the waste from the privy will drain away from the house.

In the middle of the house build a large chimney. At the base have two fireplaces, one facing into the parlor, and the other into the kitchen. During winter you will want to have both fires roaring, to keep the house warm. But even in summer keep the fires glowing as this will drive out any moisture from the walls, keeping them dry and clear. Damp walls are a major cause of every kind of disease, including fevers and aching bones.

In laying out the garden around your house, put sweet-smelling herbs near your windows; and put those herbs that are used most in cooking near the kitchen door. A little further away plant trees bearing every kind of fruit. Do not put them so near the house that their branches and leaves shade your windows. But put them near enough that you can see them from your windows. In spring their bright blossom will lift your spirits; and in autumn the sight of their succulent fruit will comfort your spirits against the prospect of winter.

In your garden dig one or two large pools, and stock them with carp. Ensure that the pools are deep, so that birds of prey cannot swoop down and eat the fish. Sitting by the pool on a warm day and watching the fish is a most pleasant way of calming the mind. And from time to time you can catch a fish for your supper.

It is now well known that air-conditioning systems can often cause illness; so some large buildings are described as sick. Andrew Boorde takes this implicit distinction between healthy and sick buildings much further, saying it should apply to almost every aspect of architecture. Even if we find ourselves doubting or disagreeing with some of his advice, his general approach raises a hugely important question: in designing and refurbishing houses, should we take physical and mental health into account, as well as utility, beauty and cost? It is hard to avoid giving an affirmative answer; and the practical implications are huge.

CHAPTER 3

MIRTHFUL SLEEPING AND WAKING

The way to ensure that you sleep soundly at night is to have ample mental and physical exercise during the day. If you are lazy in both mind and body, you will be restless and wakeful in bed. But if you are hard working and diligent, you will retire with a peaceful conscience, and will enjoy your hours of slumber. Ensure, however, that your work during the day is well balanced. If you use only your mind, - reading, writing, talking and praying - then at night you thoughts will continue to revolve in your head, and you will not sleep. So plan your routine so that you have one or two hours each day of vigorous bodily activity; this will both break the circle of your thoughts, and enable your limbs to relax.

If you wish to sleep soundly at night, there are a number of simple rules to follow. Do not go to bed in an angry or excited mood; during the hour before bed time sit quietly, reading, meditating or engaging in some simple craft such as spinning. It is best to sit in your bedroom, having lit a fire. The heat will relax your mind and body, and also expel any dampness from the air so that you will breathe easily in bed. When you go to bed open the window a little, so that fresh air mingles with the warm air, giving the ideal atmosphere for sleep. In bed do not lie on your stomach as this harms the digestion; if you feel the need for some pressure on your stomach, place your own hand there. In cold weather do not expose any bare flesh, apart from your face; ensure that the bedclothes are right up to your chin, and your arms are under the bed-clothes. Do not sleep on an empty stomach, nor on a full one; eat your evening meal one or two hours before bed time. Have two pillows under your head, so it is well above your body; this prevents feelings of nausea rising from the stomach. Put sufficient blankets on your bed so that you are warm, but not so many as to make you hot.

Sleep moderately, neither too long nor too short. Moderate sleep is good for the digestion and it nourishes the blood; it also refreshes the memory and restores the powers of the intellect. But if you allow yourself to sleep excessively, your intellect will become light and airy, and your body sluggish and watery. Excessive sleep also causes the muscles to ache and the joints to creak.

To determine how much sleep people should have one must take into account their temperament, age and strength, as well as their state of health. Those who are sanguine require seven hours sleep. Those who are choleric also need seven hours. Phlegmatic people may sleep for nine hours or more. Melancholic people are variable in their needs, sometimes sleeping for nine or ten hours, and sometimes requiring only five or six hours. Children and young people need to sleep longer at night than elderly people; but elderly people benefit from one or two naps during the day. The seasons affect the amount of sleep a person should have: add half an hour in winter, and subtract half an hour in summer.

When you undress yourself at night, sprinkle sweet-smelling herbs inside your clothes; then hang your clothes in front of the fire. So when you dress in the morning, your clothes will be fragrant and warm.

When you have risen from bed, perform various exercises that stretch your body and limbs. Bend forwards several times to touch your toes.

Twist your torso this way and that, and also your neck. Kneel down on one knee, and then the other, pushing your other leg backwards as you do so. Run on the spot, swinging your arms forward and back. All this will both fill your body with energy, and also make it feel supple and relaxed.

After you have finished your stretching exercise, dip a flannel in a bowl of water, and wipe your whole body. In the summer the water should be cold. In the winter leave the bowl by the fire overnight, so by morning it is warm. Then clean your teeth, using a brush dipped in the water.

When you have dressed, you should now take more vigorous exercise. Go for a walk, covering at least a mile; and let your pace be as fast as your legs can manage. Then use your arms, lifting up lead weights or playing bowls. It is important that your exercise is long and hard enough for your pores to open and your body to sweat. Afterwards, especially in the summer, you may now wish to undress again, and wipe yourself with cold water for a second time.

Huge numbers of us complain that we regularly do not sleep well; and the problem tends to get worse as we grow older. Much of Andrew Boorde's advice concerns sleep hygiene – the simple habits and practices that assist sound sleep – and most modern books on the subject echo Boorde's words. But he introduces an idea that is rarely now discussed: the relationship between our temperament and the amount of sleep that we need. Differences in temperament, he says, lead to huge variations in our optimal sleeping patterns. So some of us may be trying to sleep too long, and therefore merely imagine that we are suffering from insomnia. And some of us, especially those who are phlegmatic, may be endangering our health by insisting that we stay up as late as everyone else.

CHAPTER 4

MIRTHFUL EATING

The cook is the chief physician of the household. He or she is far more important to the health of the family than is the professional physician. Good food and drink, which have been wisely and skillfully prepared, are the best means of warding off disease. And the right food and drink are the best medicines for curing diseases.

If you eat day by day more food than your body needs, you will suffer all kinds of illnesses and infirmities. Your power of reason will be dulled, and your wit blunted. Your limbs will become sluggish, and even in the morning after seven or eight hours in bed you will feel tired. Your head will often ache, and your mind will be prone to wild fantasies. After many years of excessive eating your pulse will become weak and fast, and your heart will weaken. And at times you have the terrible sensation of a worm crawling round inside your body. The only cure for excessive eating is abstinence, eating less than the body needs until the body and mind are restored to health.

For most mature adults two meals a day are sufficient. For those leading sedentary lives, one meal a day may be sufficient. Only those spending their days doing hard manual labor should eat three times a day. Leave a long gap between meals; it does great damage to the stomach to add new food to food which is not fully digested. Do not linger too long at meals, as this encourages over-eating. Eat the most nutritious food at the start of the meal; so, if you feel full before the meal is complete, you can safely leave aside the less nutritious food.

Bread is the most important and nutritious food in the human diet. It may be eaten leavened or unleavened. It should be made either purely with wheat or with wheat and rye together; it is wrong to mix barley and wheat, or to put peas and beans in the bread. Bread should not be eaten when it is still hot from the oven, as it will lie on the stomach like a sponge; enjoy the smell of freshly baked bread, but do not be tempted to taste it. It is best to leave the bread in a cool larder for a day and a night before eating it.

Oats are a very nourishing grain. They may be cooked in water, with a little salt or honey, and eaten as hot porridge. Or they may be baked, with both salt and honey, and eaten as cakes.

Eggs contain much goodness, but should not be eaten in large quantities. They are easy to digest, but thicken the blood. Do not cook eggs in fat, but poach them in water, adding a little salt. They should be eaten as soon as possible after the hen has laid them; stale eggs are poisonous.

Butter in small quantities relaxes the belly, slowing the process of digestion. This has two good effects. Firstly it delays the moment when hunger returns. And secondly it enables the nutrients of other foods to be fully absorbed into the body. For these reasons butter should be eaten along with other foods during a meal; it should never be eaten separately. Butter should not, however, be eaten in large quantities. Being greasy it lies in the stomach on top of the other foods, forming a film - just as it does when added to a boiling pot. If there is excessive grease, it will block all the tubes entering the stomach, leading to indigestion and fever. Also large amounts of butter thicken the blood, which is dangerous for the liver and the heart.

Although the majority in the West has long ago ceased to do heavy manual work, we retain a pattern of meals inherited from the distant past: two, and possibly three, substantial meals a day. Small wonder that obesity is a major problem. As a monk Andrew Boorde had belonged to the small minority in medieval times that was sedentary; and he knew that a single proper meal each day is sufficient, interspersed with a few light snacks.

CHAPTER 5

MIRTHFUL DRINKING

Do not drink beer, ale, mead or wine to quench your thirst. While at first these beverages will satisfy you, they soon cause the body to become dry, so that your thirst will rage even more strongly. When you are thirsty, drink water. The purest water is rain; so collect rain from your roof in a butt. The next purest is spring water, and also water which is running fast over stones and pebbles. If neither of these is available, find a river in which you can see the bed; there should be no froth on the surface of the water, or muddy clouds within it. Only when the rivers have dried up in high summer should you drink water from a well. Water from a river or a well should be strained through a fine linen cloth before it is drunk.

When the various fruits are ripe, squeeze their juice into water, and also add honey. This makes the most delicious drink, and also quenches the thirst most effectively. For many people's palate, water flavored with strawberry and honey is the finest drink on God's earth.

To make water more pleasant to drink, you may boil it; then add chicory or the roasted roots of dandelion, and a small amount of honey. In the winter drink this concoction while it is still hot; it will warm and invigorate every part of your body. In the summer you may prefer to let it cool.

Milk from cows and ewes, especially if they have grazed on good pasture, cleanses the stomach, liver, kidneys and bowels. It also alleviates pains in the lungs and breast. But the correct quantity depends on people's temperament. A sanguine or a phlegmatic person should drink only a little milk, while a melancholic or choleric person should drink much more. Old people and children should add a little honey to their milk.

Wines may be made from grapes or from berries. Drink whichever sort you prefer. It is, however, vital that you choose your wines carefully. Wine should be clear, and not murky. It should have a pleasant smell. It should sparkle when it is poured out. It should feel cool, and not warm, in the mouth. Wine possessing all these qualities will sharpen your wits, comfort your heart, and aid your digestion.

Avoid strong red wines. These are liable to cause rheumatism, and also make the brain and the body seem heavy. In general white wine is preferable to red. Drunk in moderation white wine makes the body light and agile. The sick should drink sweet white wine.

Ale, made from malt and water, is a better drink than beer, which contains hops as well as malt and water. Beer makes a person fat, inflating the face and belly, whereas ale passes through the body easily. A good ale should be fresh and clear, rather than smokey. It should not have a film on the surface nor any dregs. The best place to store it is a cool cellar; but when it is drunk it should be slightly warm.

Posset ale, which is cold ale mixed with hot milk, is an excellent drink for those who are ill, especially those with a hot fever. Some people also recommend it as a cure for a hangover; but it is far better to avoid hangovers by drinking only moderate quantities of intoxicating beverages.

Mead, made from honey and water, is generally good for health; but people with poor digestions should avoid it. Better than mead, however, is metheglin, in which herbs are added to the honey and water. If this is clear and free from dregs, it is the most effective drink for warding off illnesses of every kind.

Do not drink beer, ale, wine and mead on an empty stomach. If you do, the liquid will go straight to your head, and so intoxicate you. The only safe drink on an empty stomach is water, with or without flavors.

Beer, wine, ale and mead should not be given to small children. The reason is that even small amounts can intoxicate a young head. Teenagers may be given these beverages diluted with water.

Pure water to quench the thirst, and a little alcohol to uplift the spirit - that is the essence of Boorde's advice on drink. This was radical in his time, since pure water was quite hard to find, and people swigged large quantities of ale on hot days – thereby dehydrating their bodies, and making themselves ill. It is equally radical today: although pure water is readily available, many people break open cans of beer on hot days.

CHAPTER 6

A MIRTHFUL BODY

Always wear linen or silk next to your skin; wool or hair irritates the skin and cause rashes. Then wear outer garments of wool or leather, according to the weather. During the winter always keep your neck warm, wearing a scarf on cold and windy days. But do not allow your head either to become too hot or too cold. So in winter wear a hat with sufficient thickness to keep away the chill, but not so thick that your head sweats. On bright, hot days in summer, wear a hat to protect your head from the rays of the sun.

As you go about your business, you will meet people with whom you wish to stop and talk. Do not stand for any length of time on stones, especially in winter, as their hard coldness will enter your feet and chill your body. Instead stand on soft grass. If there is a cold wind blowing, find shelter from it; a cold wind against a stationary body can induce the most terrible illnesses.

If possible, the sick should be given milk from a woman's breast. Since God has designed it for babies, it possesses two supreme qualities: it is digested with great ease; and it fights off illness - to which babies are especially vulnerable. These qualities make it ideal for the treatment of any disease.

The best way to build up your resistance to contagious diseases is to eat ample fruit. Pears are especially helpful; apples are also good. In the late winter, when there is no fresh fruit, drink a small cup of cider each day, possibly mixed with honey.

When there is a contagious disease in your neighbor's house, strive to keep the air in your own house pure. You an purify the air by burning juniper, rosemary, marjoram or frankincense - or a mixture of them. Also keep a fire of wood or charcoal continually burning; but ensure the smoke goes up the chimney, and not into the room.

When the skin is cut, wine should be poured on the wound. This helps to prevent the wound from becoming poisonous.

In cold weather butter should be rubbed into the chest. This helps to protect the lungs from chills.

CHAPTER 7

A MIRTHFUL MIND

Persistent tiredness, even when a person has had ample sleep, is cool and moist. So those suffering from chronic fatigue should consume things that are hot and dry. They should fry or roast their meat and vegetables, eating them as soon as they are cooked; and they should add pepper and other spices to their food. When they eat fruit, they should sprinkle it with ginger. They should also eat ample mint. The leaves may be added to food in the later stages of cooking; but, better still, they may be boiled in water, and the water drunk.

Anxiety is hot and moist. So suffering from undue anxiety, even about quite trivial matters, should reduce it by consuming things that are cool and dry. They should roast or braise their meat and vegetables, rather than boiling them or frying them; and before eating them, they should let the meat and vegetables become tepid or even cold. Apart from salt they should avoid adding extra flavors to their food; bland food is an excellent cure for anxiety. They should drink wine rather than ale, and white wine rather than red. Herbs for easing anxiety include chamomile, lavender, rosemary and St John's wort.

Anger is hot and dry. So those suffering from excessive anger should overcome it by consuming things that are cool and moist. They should boil their meat; but where possible they should eat their vegetables raw. They should avoid all red meat, preferring the meat of poultry to that of animals. They should prefer white wine to red; and ale is better than mead. They should have herbs that cool the brain and moisten the body: fumitory, wormwood and centaury are especially valuable. They should also eat ample fruit, especially rhubarb.

Depression is cold and dry. So those suffering from depression should overcome it by consuming things that are hot and moist. They should boil their meat and vegetables in water, rather than frying them. They should flavor their food with pepper, and use a minimum amount of salt. They should drink sweet wine and mead, and avoid bitter wines and ale. They should also have herbs that bring heat and moisture to the body and brain: borage, marjoram and thyme are especially recommended

While many aspects of modern medical treatment, such as surgery, have become hugely sophisticated, and often highly effective, the treatment of mental illness remains crude. And in recent times there have been several new drugs that were initially hailed as wonder-cures, and then later turned out to have very damaging long-term consequences. Andrew Boorde's analysis of mental problems in terms of humidity and temperature is hard to justify in scientific terms; but this does not necessarily discredit the dietary prescriptions that arise from it. If and when we suffer from any of the problems that he mentions, we can simply ask ourselves: does his dietary advice feel right? If so, we can do ourselves no harm by following it, and may do ourselves great good.